hathayoga

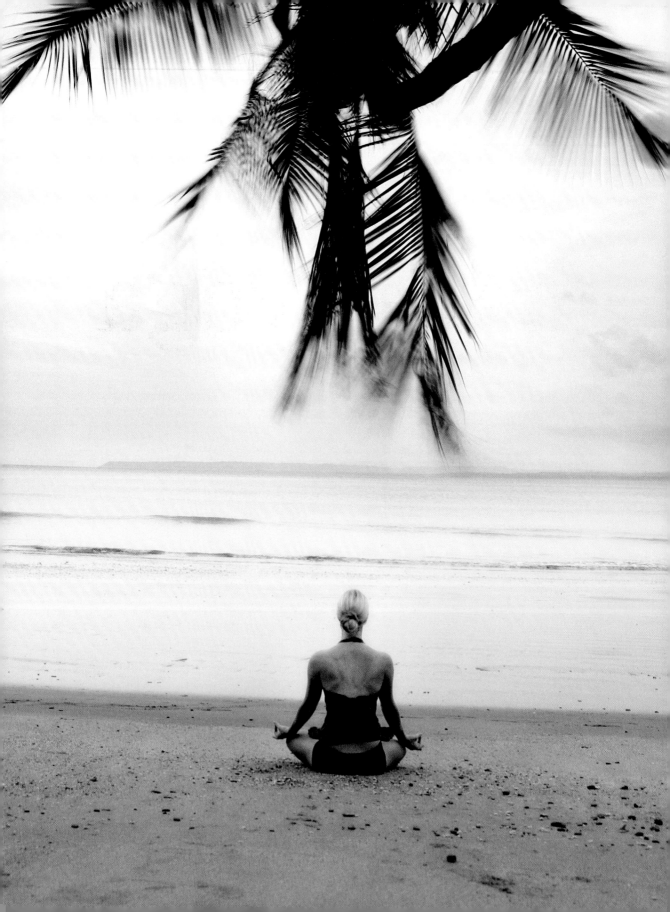

hatha yoga

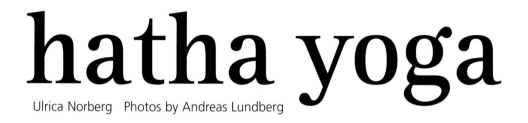

Ulrica Norberg   Photos by Andreas Lundberg

Skyhorse Publishing

Skyhorse Publishing books may be purchased in bulk at special discounts for sales promotion, corporate gifts, fund-raising, or educational purposes. Special editions can also be created to specifications. For details, contact the Special Sales Department, Skyhorse Publishing, 555 Eighth Avenue, Suite 903, New York, NY 10018 or info@skyhorsepublishing.com.

www.skyhorsepublishing.com

Library of Congress Cataloging-in-Publication Data

Norberg, Ulrica.
  [Hathayoga. English]
  Hatha yoga : the body's path to balance, focus, and strength / Ulrica
Norberg ; photos by Andreas Lundberg.
       p. cm.
  Includes bibliographical references and index.
  ISBN-13: 978-1-60239-218-2 (pbk. : alk. paper)
  ISBN-10: 1-60239-218-8 (pbk. : alk. paper)
  1. Hatha yoga. I. Title.

RA781.7N66613 2008
613.7'046--dc22

                                                    2007041159

10 9 8 7 6 5 4 3 2

Printed in the United States of America

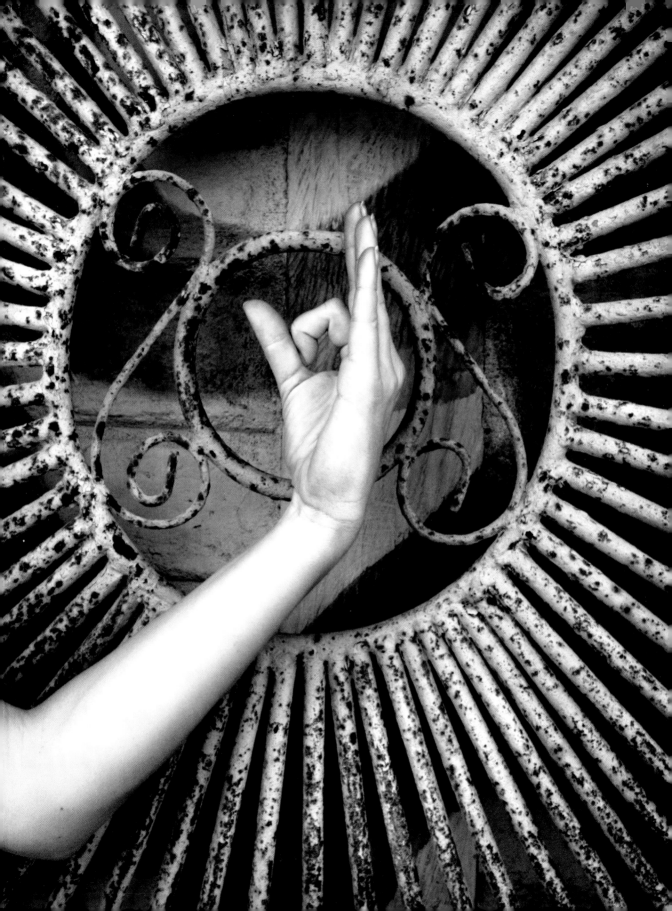

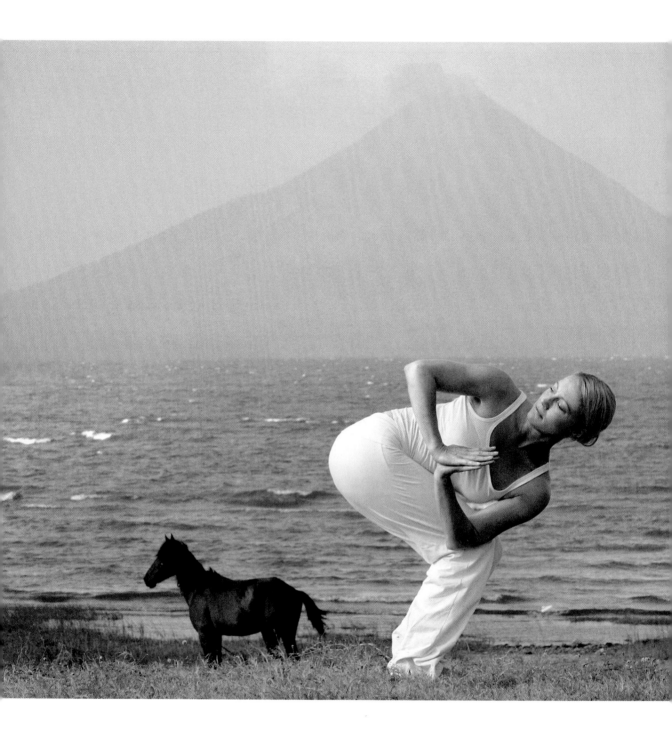

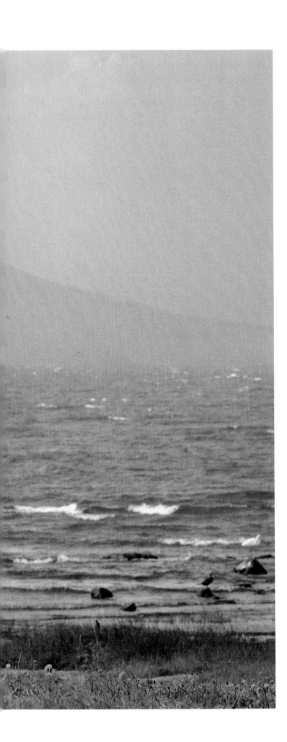

contents

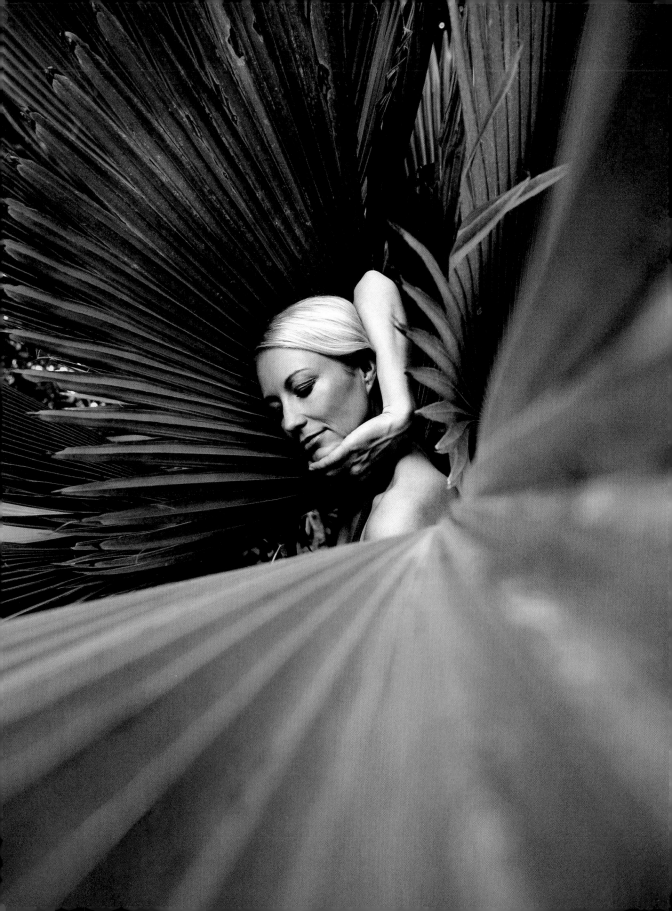

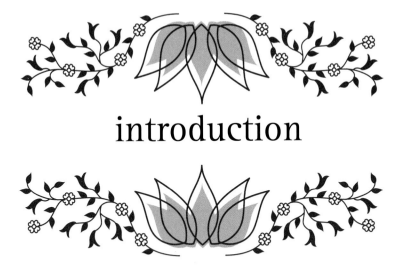

introduction

Yoga is balance (samatva). — *Bhagavad Gita (2.48)*

The ancient Indian practice of yoga has become incredibly popular today, with the number of new practitioners growing daily. One reason for the great interest in this extremely venerated practice is that it creates a great path for personal growth and an opportunity to increase awareness, strength, and relaxation.

The world has always been demanding for human beings, for one reason or another. To meet the challenges we are faced with, we've been forced to find ways to survive and develop the energy needed to get through each day. The ancient text *Bhagavad Gita* describes the world as a battlefield, where it is crucial to hold onto functioning morals and ethics. At the same time, people must reflect on their norms and values so that they—and their surroundings—can thrive in each situation while maintaining the natural, the noble, and the good. It's pretty much the same today; to be happy and feel good in life we need to be in harmony with ourselves and with our surroundings. It is here that yoga offers the opportunity to strengthen ourselves and to grow both as individuals and as a species.

To a great degree yoga is about life, life force, and how to reach our maximum potential as human beings. The techniques of yoga are designed to bring increased awareness and harmony, both within and without, for the individual who practices them on a regular basis. When we accept our own nature and improve our health, we also create lasting and harmonious surroundings and communities, instead of discarding them the minute they aren't convenient. Morals, ethics, communication, reflection, and respect for life are essential elements that enlightened people in northern India realized early on were essential for growth as a group and for individuals to reach their full potential. Still today we struggle with maintaining tranquility, peace, harmony, and our world.

To practice yoga means to always be present in the moment, in everything you do, and to act from a self-awareness and an awareness of the outer world, with the goal of finding joy, happiness, and harmonious development. It requires training as well as discipline and reflection. You have to take one step at a time. Hatha Yoga is a way to good health and universal well-being.

This book is an attempt at a comprehensive presentation of classic Hatha Yoga with its various elements. It is not easy to fully explain physical yoga's roots and to show the yogic way the respect it deserves all in one book. We were thus forced to limit ourselves; so we decided to give preference to the asanas—what they consist of and how to position the body—since it is this dimension we often come in contact with first in yoga. The other aspects we've highlighted on a smaller scale. By no means do I mean to imply that asanas are the most important or leading part of yoga. But you have to start somewhere. Working with the body, breath, and focus is a good way to begin.

Producing Hatha Yoga were: Ulrica Norberg (concept/copy), Andreas Lundberg (photography), Alexandra Frank (design), and Lars-Erik Carlsson (editor). We have tried to come up with a richly illustrated book that we hope you experience as relevant, inspiring, and enriching. This book is intended for all, independent of previous experience with yoga, but above all it is meant for those that are curious and want to know more about Hatha Yoga. However, this book isn't meant as a substitute for a yoga teacher who can give individual instruction and guidance.

My advice to anyone just entering the world of yoga is to have an open mind while reflecting on this philosophy, even if some of the ideas seem complex, challenging, and even difficult for the time being. You do not have to agree. Just reflect on what is said and give it a try.

Om Shanti,
Ulrica

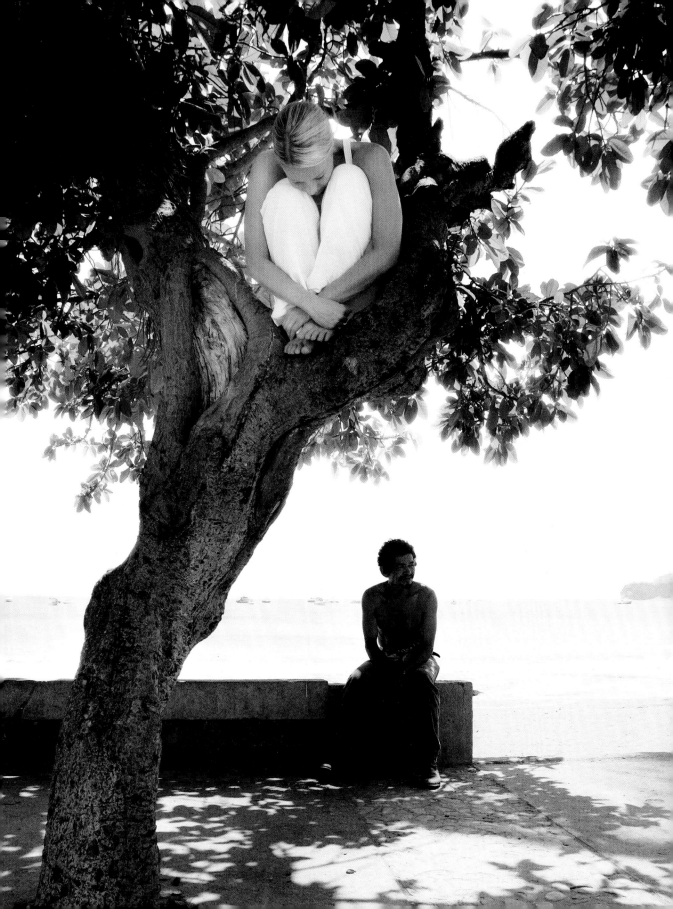

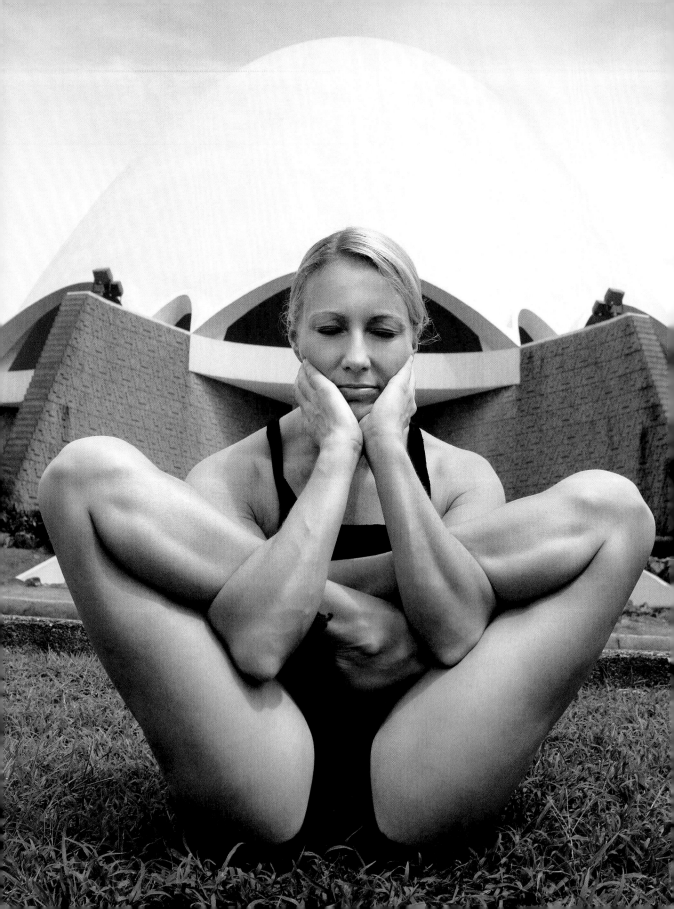

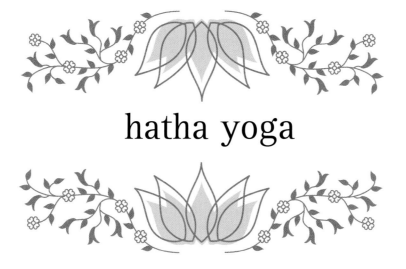

hatha yoga

Neither through action or by abstinence from action does one achieve peace; nor by renunciation alone can one attain perfection. — Bhagavad Gita (3.5)

To clarify what yoga really is, we can start with looking at what it *isn't*.

Yoga isn't a religion, cult, or New Age fad. It's not a modern fitness regime that takes a little here and a little there from Asian or Indian training systems. Yoga isn't a lifestyle choice with some predetermined number of values which must be adhered to. You don't need to light incense or wear spiritual necklaces to practice yoga. You don't need to believe in any god or live a religious life. Yoga doesn't require any blind faith, specific prerequisites, or knowledge. There also aren't any requirements for penance or confession, humiliation, or self-denial. You don't have to give up any specific food, alcohol, sex, or money. You don't have to be nimble, young, rich, skinny, beautiful, or trendy. You only have to be yourself, just as you are. The only things yoga recommends are moderation, openness, and regular reflection about what is happening inside you.

The word "yoga" has a broad meaning. The basic definition is "yoke, join, unify" in Sanskrit. Yoga is about joining together two dimensions; humanity (brahman) and an individual's true self (atman) to find balance between the two.

13

Yoga's historical background

Yoga is one of six schools of thought that together are called *Darsana* (the way to see). These can be seen as different perspectives on how life, living, and energy work together in different ways in time and space as well as outside and inside every living thing. That which distinguishes yoga from the other schools of thought is that it deals entirely with human potential. Yoga highlights and even describes the methods that can increase life force and harmonious development in life. All the techniques deal with insights and wisdom about humans and their nature.

Yoga is not one tradition but the result of many traditions that overlapped each other and between which there was even some exchange. In any case, yoga is still completely vibrant today and is still developing, especially in the western world. Yogic philosophy has developed through wisdom and experience and has thus kept pace with society's needs and changes. That's why you'll find a different approach in the east than in the west. New dimensions of yoga are attributed to different encounters with novel environments and peoples, but the principles remain the same. This is what is fascinating about yoga—that it is so enduring. One of my first yoga teachers said to me that what keeps yoga so strong is that in the end it concentrates on the essence of life and what is human. As she went on to say: "There is only one truth but many roads to reach it."

To develop deeper insight and knowledge of yoga, it is helpful to read the history and philosophy from the ancient yogic literature such as the *Vedas*, *Upanishads*, the *Bhagavad Gita*, and *Yoga Sutra*.

Yoga sutra—the source of yogic understanding

The Sanskrit text *Yoga Sutra*'s 196 aphorisms or verses point to a method that can help yoga practitioners strengthen mind, body, and soul. *Yoga Sutra* describes the royal path of yoga, *Raja Yoga*, as a meditative yogic path to happiness and harmony in life through strengthening and balancing the mind. *Raja Yoga* incorporates *Karma Yoga* (deeds and destiny), *Bhakti Yoga* (devotion and humility), *Jnana Yoga* (knowledge/wisdom), and *Kriya Yoga* (active, cleansing deeds and exercises). *Yoga Sutra* is considered by many yogis to be the heart of yoga and the source of yogic understanding. *Yoga Sutra*'s author, Patanjali, defines yoga as "yoga citta vritti nirodah," which can be translated as "yoga is the ability to direct the mind exclusively towards an object and sustain focus in that direction without any distractions." Practicing yoga means striving for a balanced mental state, which with training strengthens you in every way. These techniques encompass everything from our attitude and values to how we eat, sleep, and function in daily life. Mental stress leading to imbalance can express itself in different ways: we can have physical pain, or feel spiritually lost or mentally worn out.

Yoga Sutra is divided into four books (chapters) called Padas. These are *Samadhi Pada*, which describes what yoga is; *Vibhuti Pada*, which discusses the hurdles that stand in yoga's way; and *Kaivalya Pada*, which talks about how to free yourself from what leads you to imbalances. In *Sadhana Pada*, Patanjali describes the eight roads: *Yama, Niyama, Asana, Pranayama, Pratyahara, Dharana, Dhyana, Samadhi*.

Yama, Niyama, Asana, and Pranayama are physical paths. These come from our own effort, training, and actions. Dharana, Dhyana, and Samadhi are subtler paths. These paths, or phases in development, just "happen" as a result of the first four paths. Pratyahara is the balance between them, the bridge between the physical paths and the "mental" paths, and is a requirement for Dharana, concentration, to arise. The first two halves of this eight-fold path, Yama and Niyama, include a type of preparatory moral to inspire the yogi/yogini. It is an ethical base on which everything is built, but is complex and impossible to slavishly follow, which would defeat the purpose anyway. Each individual is unique and should find his or her own balance.

Asanas and pranayama are about how we treat our bodies and how we breathe or manage our energy as individuals. Pratyahara deals with focus, being present, and teaching us to turn our mental awareness inward and turn down the mental activity, similar to turning down the stereo. We turn the awareness inward and observe what happens in body and mind. Dharana means concentration. Here it means to try to fix all our awareness toward a specific thing or goal, without letting the focus drift away. Dhyana, meditation, is a branch of Dharana and includes a deeper state of concentration. Samadhi is often described as a serene state in which you recognize your self, who you truly are: a process or a condition in which the meditator gets completely engaged in the meditation.

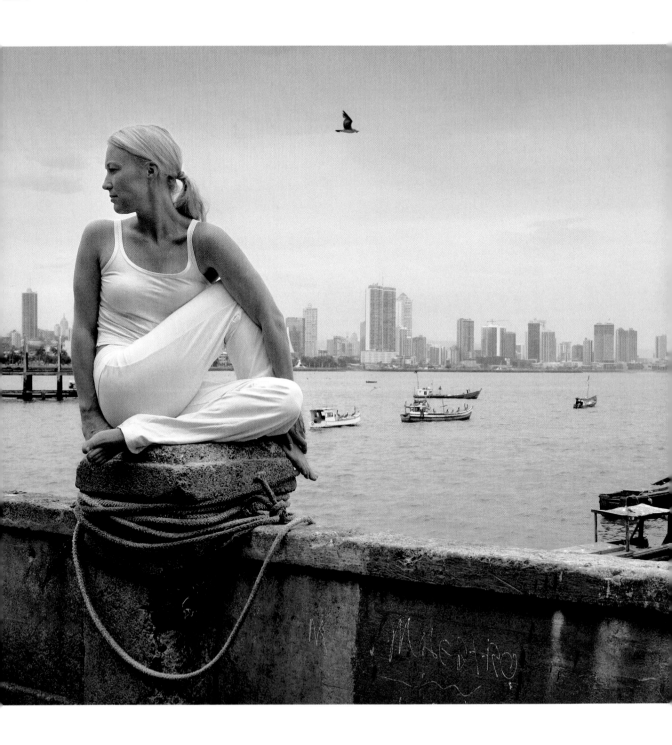

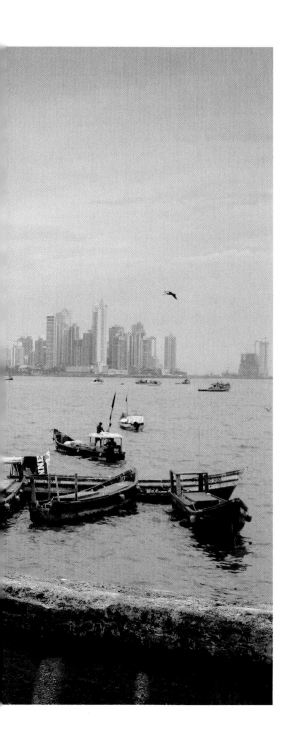

Hatha Yoga

Hatha Yoga is considered the youngest of yoga's six primary forms and descends, as the other forms do, from *Tantra Yoga* (teachings on energy), the oldest yoga form. The other branches are *Karma Yoga* (teachings on action), *Bhakti Yoga* (teachings on devotion), *Jnana Yoga* (teachings on knowledge), and *Raja Yoga* (teachings on mental awareness). These different paths demonstrate the development of yoga over thousands of years. They can be seen as the various yogic fields of study, separate practices and perspectives on ways of life.

Hatha Yoga has its roots in medieval Indian philosophy. Different from early yoga traditions, where the primary focus was on meditation, here the body plays a larger role. As Hatha Yoga developed, experiments began in physical training (asanas) as well as with different breathing techniques (pranayama), due to the thought that the body must be strong before the mind can be disciplined. It developed into the practice of self-discipline and physical control.

The word *hatha* means forceful, but it is also a conjunction of two words, *ha*, which means sun, and *tha*, which means moon in ancient Sanskrit. The joining together of these two polarities hints at yoga's purpose: to find balance both within and without, in this case between two universal energy forms—the solar, contracting energy and the lunar, expanding energy. These two energy forms are worked with in different ways in order to release physical and psychic blockages, stress, and tension, and instead to build strength, endurance, and life-giving power so the thoughts may be stilled while the body relaxes. This leads to increased self-knowledge and self-confidence. We become united with the inner source of power that all of us have within ourselves.

When we practice asanas we combine and balance the masculine and feminine energy within each of us, whether we are a man or a woman. According to Hatha Yoga philosophy, each individual must begin by balancing the physical body so that the mind can also be strengthened. If the body is strong, it creates a counterweight and positively influences mental power. But the mind also must be strengthened so that it, in its turn, can strengthen the body. These two function in harmony. If the mind and body are weak, the soul is more easily influenced and wounded. Psychic-physical yoga movements lead to a calm, focused mind and a strong and flexible body and bring a feeling of wholeness, harmony, freedom, and peace to the soul.

In *Yoga Sutra*, yoga asanas are defined as *Stirham sukham asanam*, "Asanas must have the dual qualities of alertness and relaxation." This is important because the body must be strengthened so the practitioner can sit in the same position for a long period without losing awareness because the body is giving out. Yoga asanas are thus a preparation for meditation.

Hatha Yoga positions are divided into different types of asanas (body positions), pranayama (breath control), Raj asanas (meditative positions), and Nauli, Mudras, and Bandhas (cleaning and clearing positions).

There are a vast number of different forms of Hatha Yoga today. The most well-known varieties are Ananda Yoga, Bikram Yoga, Kundalini Yoga, Kripalu Yoga, Sivananda Yoga, Vini Yoga, Power Yoga (Vinyasa Yoga), Iyengar Yoga, and Ashtanga Vinyasa Yoga. My advice to you is if you have found a form that you enjoy, stay with it awhile. If eventually you feel that you want to discover other dimensions of Hatha Yoga, the possibilities are endless.

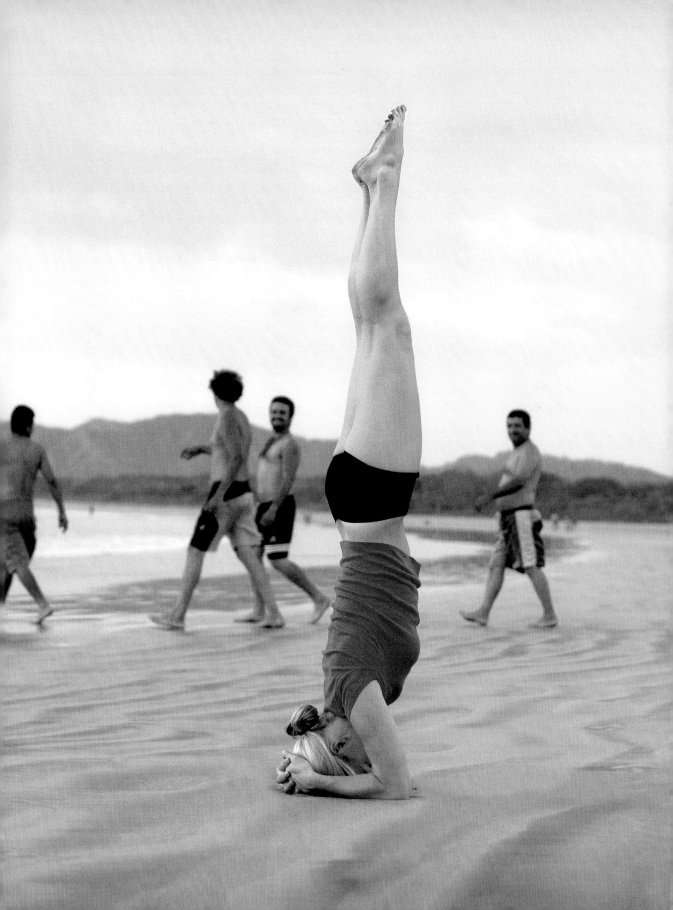

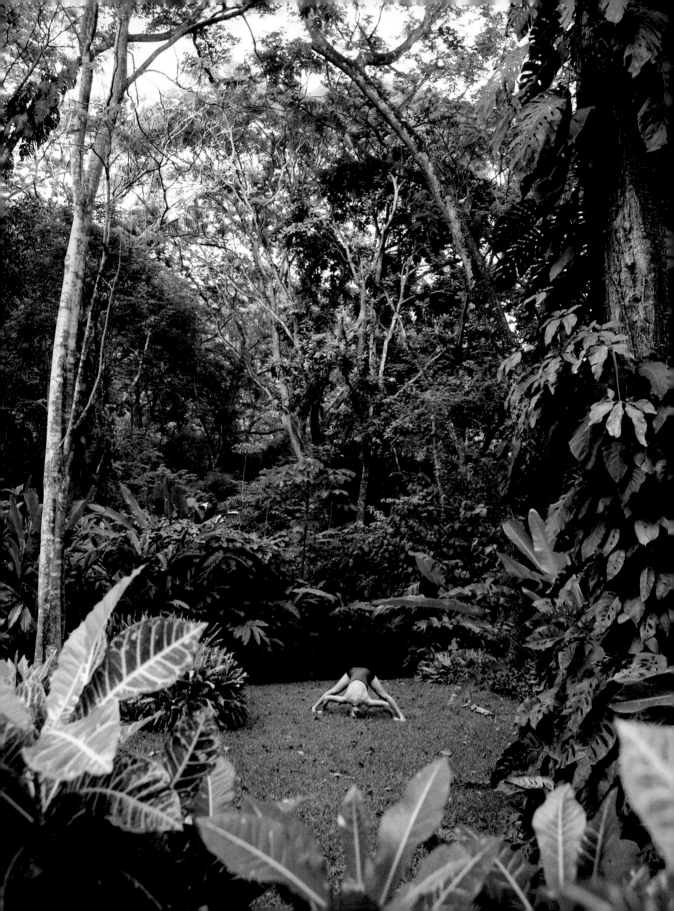

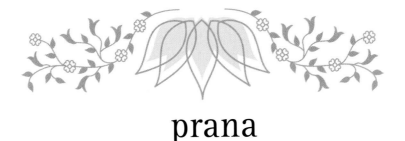

prana

The embodied spirit, master of the city of his body, does not create activities,
nor does he induce people to act, nor does he create the fruits of action.
All this is enacted by the modes of material nature.
—*Bhagavad Gita 5.14*

Hatha Yoga can be seen as a way to release energy locked in the body by practicing physical forms (asanas) that together with breath awareness lead to increased blood circulation. These movements recharge us with new power and make us feel stronger, more alert, and more harmonious. We expand the possibilities to receive and develop vitality. This verve or life force is called *prana* in Sanskrit. Hatha Yoga's techniques strengthen us physically, mentally, and spiritually.

Prana links together the body (material) with the soul (non-material) and streams out through the body via what are called *nadis* (channels that originate along the spine), giving energy to the body's organs and cells. Prana's river creates energy fields that vibrate or circulate at different frequencies, depending upon how much energy is entering that path. The paths are called *chakras*.

Chakra, which means "wheel" in Sanskrit and "light circle" in Hindu, can be seen as a system of generators that regulate, store, and support the body with prana, vitality. These chakras are zones in the body where different *nadis* meet. According to yogic philosophy there are 72,000 nadis in the body. There are three central ones: *Sushumma Nadi* (corresponding to the central nervous system), *Ida Nadi*, and *Pingala Nadi* (corresponding to the autonomous nervous system).

The chakra system seems to many to be difficult to understand and rather odd and complex. In the end it isn't so hard. Thousands of years before modern medicine entered our daily lives with its theories, yogic philosophy offered an enormous amount of knowledge and wisdom about people and how they work and behave. The chakra system is an ancient method for describing the complexity of how our nervous systems, minds, muscles, and organs function and describes how everything inside and outside us are connected. Chakras can be seen as databases that contain information we can't get from the physical world. These databases contain information about everything concerning ourselves, including thoughts, instincts, memories, etc.

Through the different movements in yoga we stimulate the different chakras. We have seven inside the body and five above and outside the body. The physical chakras correspond to our nerve center, the solar plexus. These are the *Muladhara chakra* (root chakra), *Svadistana chakra* (genital chakra), *Manipura chakra* (navel chakra), *Anahata chakra* (heart chakra), *Vishuddhi chakra* (throat chakra), *Ajna chakra* (third eye), and *Sahasrara chakra* (crown chakra).

Tension and stress in the body are released through energy streams beginning to flow with the breath, as well as through standing positions and physical movements, asanas. Hatha Yoga deals with power, refining the life energy both within and without each individual. The more prana one has flowing in the body, the more balanced, positive, and strong one becomes.

Can you increase prana?

The amount of prana is finite and can't be increased or decreased. So when we say that we increase prana in the body and mind we mean that we change the energy that is already available to a creative, positive force, which makes it possible for us to grow and develop.

The first step to increasing prana in the body is to practice deep and conscious breathing. Concentrated breathing promotes mental and physical health in many ways: first by increasing the intake of oxygen and energy, and then through conscious concentration, which brings us more into the present. It calms that which in yoga is referred to as "monkey mind;" a mental state that's compared to a monkey who restlessly hops from tree to tree with no particular goal.

Prana's five dimensions

The following five dimensions (winds, or *vayus*, as they are also called) are different ways to describe how prana is distributed in the body. They function both as a whole and as distinct units in the body. If an imbalance occurs in one unit it is compensated for in another, which is often a big contributor to unevenness in the body.

Prana vayus = Rising breath (the positive interpretation of prana). This prana lives in the heart, is light and energy-giving and associated with fire and sun energy. In contrast to the universal power with the same name, this individualized prana comes up through the *pingala nadi* on the right side of the spinal column and looks after the chest (from the diaphragm to the throat), midriff, and belly. It controls speech, throat, and breath as well as blood circulation and the muscles and nerves that activate this region. This is the energy that helps prana move through the atmosphere into the body.

Apana vayus = Falling breath (the negative interpretation of prana). *Apana*, which means "the energy that lives below," lives under the belly button and distributes energy to the lower half of the body, specifically the largest internal organs, the intestines, the anus, and the genitals. Apana vayus works at eliminating waste, toxins, and negative energy from the body. Its character is calming and centering; it is associated with the moon and controls exhalation.

Samana vayus = Nourishing breath. *Samana* consists of two conjoined words. *Sam*, which means "together," and *an*, which means "to breathe." Samana distributes energy in the form of nourishment, *rasa*, and moves it through the body to create power and energy. Samana runs through all limbs and is responsible for bodily functions such as food burning and for the liver, the small intestine, and the pancreas and its secretions (insulin). Samana activates the heart and the respiratory system. Earlier texts have placed this center in the heart, but Hatha Yoga texts put it in the navel.

Udana vayus = Up breath. *Udana* means "up" in Sanskrit and refers to the region above the neck. Udana provides the eyes, the nose, and the ears with energy. Consciousness of the outside world would be impossible without this energy. Udana *vayus* sends life energy out toward the extremities and their muscles, joints, ligaments, and nerves, supports the stomach region with energy, and is responsible for maintaining good posture through the spine.

Vyana vayus = Diffuse breath. *Vyana* means "wind" and is present throughout the body in each cell. Vyana regulates and controls all movement and coordinates all the other prana forces. It is also kept as a reserve energy source to use if the other vayus are imbalanced. Vyana principally sends energy to the limbs, eyes, ears, and the throat and supports the intake of prana and the exhalation of apana. Some older texts claim that *vyana vayus* activates facility of speech and articulation.

Prana and lifestyle

Our lifestyle has a huge effect on these different pranas. Physical activity, what we eat, and our sexual relationships influence the circulation and flow of prana in the body. Feelings, thoughts, and fantasies are even more influential. An irregular and unbalanced lifestyle, bad diet, and negative stress can prevent, impede, or significantly reduce prana in the body. This

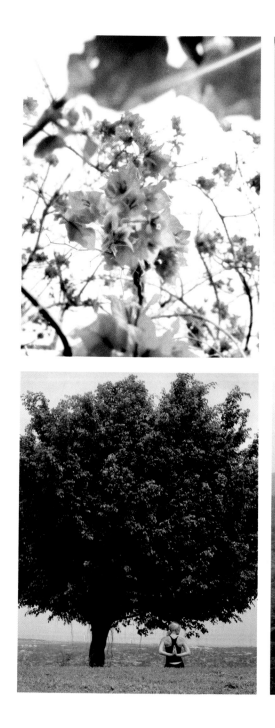

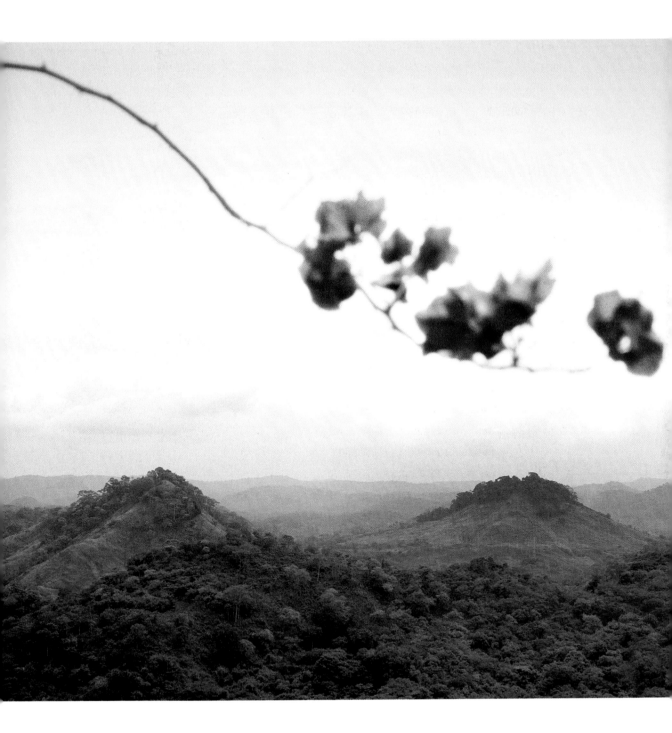

results, according to yogic thought, in feeling drained. If prana is nearly emptied from a specific chakra, it can lead to sickness and imbalance in overall metabolic functioning. Pranayama techniques (see page 39) work to restore our balance and can control energy so it isn't depleted. Pranayama exercises are recommended before and after asanas.

Yoga asanas and prana

Prana is circulating in the entire body and follows set pathways, which are responsible for how cell activity happens inside us. Stiffness in the body is a result of blocked prana, often due to constant absorption of toxins. When prana flows again, the toxins are released and sloughed off from the places where they earlier were hidden, raising overall health throughout the body. This means that positions that were once impossible to master may suddenly seem inviting and very doable. In addition, posture, balance, strength, and agility are noticeably improved.

Yoga asanas and kundalini

Yoga is said to awaken *kundalini*, primordial power, our hidden potential. Conscious control over kundalini opens and deepens consciousness and provides insights and spiritual experiences far beyond ordinary consciousness. This often starts with a need to meditate and intensify the contact with our inner store of wisdom. Through increased contact with this spiritual energy, a larger understanding of other dimensions is awakened. Kundalini is often described as a small snake lying coiled and sleeping at the base of the spine. The goal is to awaken the snake so that it uncoils and brings our life force out of hiding. Kundalini is a concentrate of the universal life energy, a part of ourselves but at the same time something much larger. Or to say it another way, kundalini is not energy; instead energy is a byproduct of kundalini.

When kundalini is awakened, a large surge of prana is released and quickly rises through Sushumna nadi to activate all of our chakras. When our chakras are open and Sushumna nadi is unblocked, kundalini is free to rise. Unfortunately, sometimes this power is awakened in individuals who aren't properly prepared, who may still have large blockages in their chakras. The results can be unexpected pain (most often in the back), shakiness, hot flashes, light and sound hallucinations, extreme sensitivity, hyperactivity . . .

the list is long. It isn't just through yoga that kundalini can be awakened without the necessary readiness. Kundalini can also be spontaneously activated, either awakened or put to sleep, without our own conscious involvement.

Through working with asanas we influence the different chakras that are intended to move kundalini around the entire body. There are approximately thirty-five asanas aimed at specific chakras. The other asanas are aimed at cleansing and regulating the nadis so that they may take up and transport prana through the body. The chief purpose of Hatha Yoga is to create a balance between the pranic and the mental energies in the body. This leads to a release of tension and stress from the body and brings an upsurge of strength, freedom, and vitality. This energy can remain in the body, sometimes throughout our lifetime, sometimes for shorter periods in the various chakras. In Hatha Yoga the purpose of the movements, the poses, and the breathing techniques is to awaken these energies, which can be the beginning of increased awareness and attention to one's self as well as to others. Hatha Yoga is devised so that kundalini isn't awakened before the body and the mind are well prepared, strong, and balanced. In practice, beginners probably won't be thinking about either the flow of prana or kundalini energy, which is how it should be. Instead, they should keep practicing awareness, which will lead to increased insight, knowledge, and understanding.

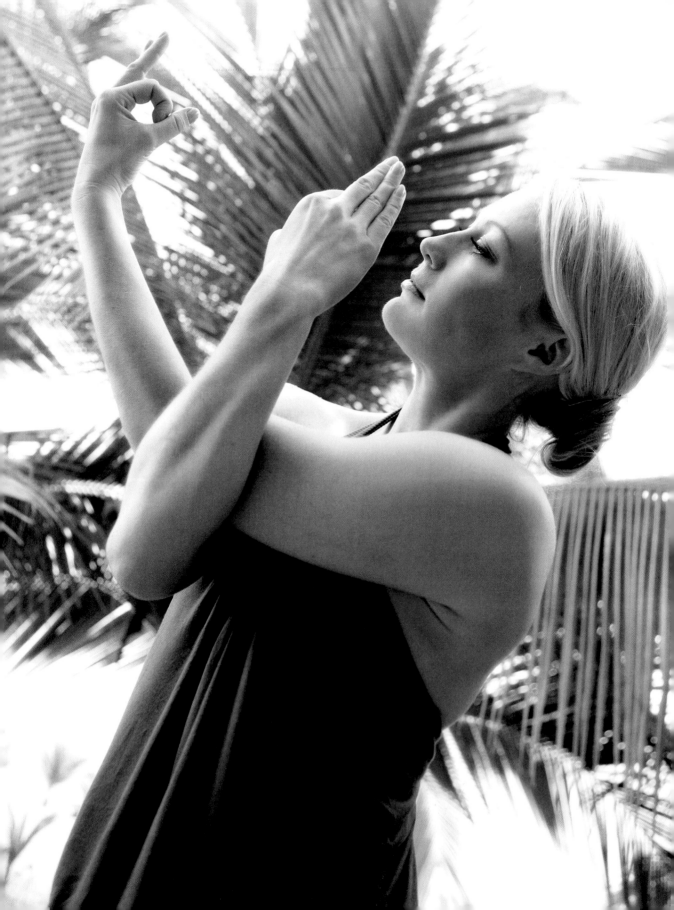

mudras, drishti, and bandhas

Mudras are a combination of movements that can direct energy for our moods, physical poses, and our awareness and powers of observation. Practicing mudras results in increased concentration and consciousness.

A mudra can include the entire body in a combination of asanas, pranayama, bandhas, and visualization techniques, or it can be as simple as a hand movement. The yoga text *Hathayoga Pradipika* defines mudras as a *yoganga*, an independent branch of yoga involved with training and developing the psyche through physical and sensory training.

Mudras work with prana by directing it through the body, for the prana that exists in the body is by nature outgoing. In this way we steer the outgoing and the internal energies so that they meet, which is a continuation of energy development. There are five different types of yoga mudras, but mostly they are hand and head mudras. Below we give an explanation of the five mudra groups. I have concentrated on the first group because they are used so much more often and to a fuller extent in asanas and pranayama than the other groups.

Hasta: hand mudras

Hand mudras are often presented as meditative mudras. Here we use different placements of the hands and the fingers in order to train the nervous system in different ways (on pages 31-33 you can find various *hasta* mudras).

Mana: head mudras

These are common in kundalini yoga as well as the more meditative purposes in Raja and Hatha Yoga. Different head mudras are used to train the eyes, the ears, the nose, the tongue, and the lips.

Kaya: posture mudras

These mudras are aimed at training and developing the postural muscles (both in the back and in the legs). By practicing these, which include physical poses in combination with breathing and concentration, you will improve and create more awareness around your posture. Asanas also play a role in posture, but Kaya mudras should be practiced first as posture, a prerequisite for good technique during asanas.

Mudra bandha: "lock" mudras

These combine mudra and bandha. Bandhas recharge the body with prana, greatly strengthening the muscles of the trunk, among other things. The inner organs are oxygenated, thanks to increased circulation, and prepared for kundalini awakening. Read more about the bandhas on page 34.

Adhara: perineal "lock," inner muscle contraction/extension training

This technique coordinates prana from the body to the brain. This works primarily with strengthening the entire area around the pelvic bowl, the belly, and the loins to achieve a security in the body as well as the mind and the nervous system, so individuals can continue developing.

Hasta mudra: hand positions

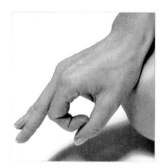

Jnana mudra: the gesture of knowledge

Jnana means wisdom and intuitive knowledge. Jnana mudra is a method for cultivating inner wisdom.

Sit in a relaxed position. Bend the index finger so that it reaches to the inside of the base of the thumb (it is common for the thumb and the index finger to touch). Stretch the other fingers, holding them gently apart and keeping them relaxed. Place the hands on the knees, palms of the hands facing down. Relax the arms and the hands. Sitting in Ardha Padmasana (half-lotus) pose while the hands are in jnana mudra and focusing on breathing is one of the most common starting points for asanas, meditation, and pranayama practice, as it is an excellent way to increase concentration, focus, and relaxation.

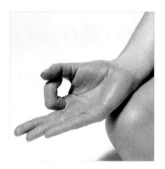

Chin mudra: the gesture of consciousness

Chin comes from the word chit, or chitta, which means consciousness. This mudra helps to cultivate consciousness.

Chin mudra is done in the exact same fashion as Jnana mudra except that the palms of the hands are facing up instead of down. Sitting in Ardha Padmasana with Chin mudra and breathing deeply is a common way to end practice. If you've already started in sitting position with Jnana mudra, you will experience a greater sense of calm. By ending your asana session in the same way you began, you will find increased stability and inner security.

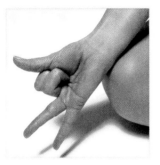

Hridaya mudra: heart gesture

Hridaya means heart, and this mudra helps to manifest and stabilize the emotions. This hand gesture is also called Vishnu mudra.

Sit in a comfortable position, with the neck and back in a straight line. Lay the hands on the knees with the palms of the hands facing up. Come into Chin mudra with the right hand. Then move the right index finger and middle finger in towards the base of the thumb and gently stretch out the other two fingers (this mudra is used in Nadi Shodhana, see page 45, with the right hand turned upwards and in some other pranayama practices with the left hand turned upwards). Relax, close the eyes and try to find stillness.

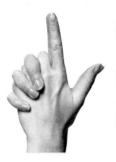

Yoni mudra: gesture of your source

Yoni means source as well as womb. Yoni mudra is said to awaken feelings of self-assuredness and self-confidence.

Interlacing the fingers in this gesture creates circulation that binds the right and left hands and even the two sides of the body. This mudra balances the energy in the body and between the two sides of the brain. Yoni mudra helps to increase physical balance in asanas and gives a higher level of concentration, relaxation, and consciousness. The elbows should point a bit outwards, still relaxed, when you do this mudra, to help open the chest area.

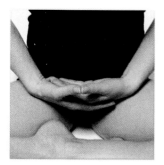

Bhairavi mudra: power gesture

Bhairava means powerful and intense. Bhairavi mudra is used foremost in meditation and pranayama.

Sit in a comfortable position, keeping the spine and the neck in a straight line. Place the back of the left hand into the palm of the right hand (*Bhairavi*). Relax, close the eyes, and practice stillness. Imagine that you are releasing all that you no longer need through the navel down into the hands. When the right hand rests in the left hand it is called *Bhairava mudra*, being the masculine counterpart of the feminine *Bhairavi*.

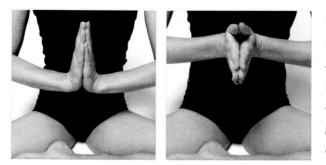

Anjali mudra: gesture of greeting

Also called the Namaskara mudra. Anjali means sealing and Namaskara means respectful greeting. Anjali mudra is a gesture for balance and harmony.

This mudra balances the energy between the body and the soul, the right and left sides of the body, the right and left sides of the brain, etc. This is a uniting gesture and stabilizes the body while expressing self-respect and respect for others around you.

Drishti

Each of the asanas has one or more specific *drishti*, or focusing points. This facilitates (and is a prerequisite for) good posture. Applying drishti helps to focus the mind inward and provides counterbalance to the posture itself. This inner focus develops *Pratyahara (focus)* and *Dharana* (concentration) and *Dhyana* (meditation), the sixth and seventh steps of the eight-fold yogic path.

The ten most common drishtis are: *Nasagrai* (looking at the tip of the nose); *Angusta ma d'ya* (looking at the thumb or at a specific finger); *Broomadhya* (looking toward the third eye, between the eyebrows); *Nabi* (looking in toward the navel, not directly at it but toward it); *Urdhva* (looking up, toward the sky); *Hastagrai* (looking up toward or at the right or left hand); *Padhayoragrai* (looking down toward or at the toes); *Maya drishti* (looking at the periphery); and *Parsva*, sometimes called *Prasva* (looking out to the left horizon or looking in to the right horizon).

Bandhas

Bandha means lock in Sanskrit and involves engaging the inner musculature of the trunk. The purpose of these exercises is to give support to the spine and the inner organs during asanas. They contribute to maintaining warmth in the body during practice and to stabilizing the pulse and neutralizing brain activity. They can be used as simple postural training by sitting in *Padmasana* (Lotus pose), standing in *Tadasana* (Mountain pose), or lying in *Shavasana* (Corpse pose). They work with pelvic floor strengthening, core stability, and posture specifically in the upper body, hips, throat, and neck. They can even be integrated into pranayama techniques to bring about better posture, increased heat and circulation in the body, increased breath capacity, and a higher level of focus and deep concentration. Bandhas are also an obvious part of asana training, as they create a support for the belly, the trunk, the pelvis, and the back so that the vertebral column isn't overstrained. In addition, bandhas are one of the requirements for holding the spine in proper position while executing some of the different asanas.

There are three different types of bandhas that are integrated in yoga training. They are *Mula bandha, Uddiyana bandha*, and *Jalandhara bandha*.

Mula banda: root lock. Pulling up through the pelvic musculature, tighten and lift

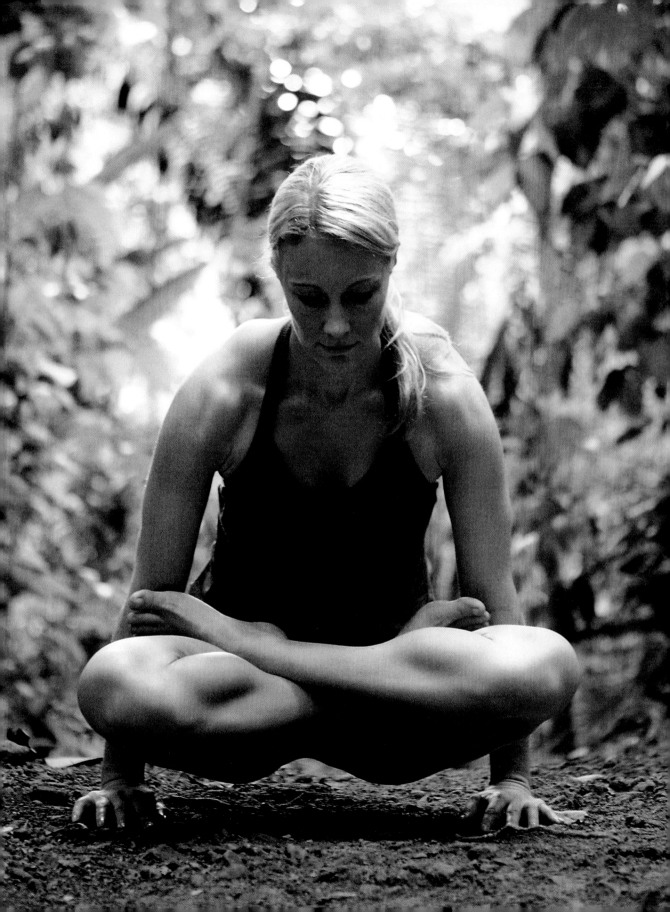

the perineum, which lies between the genitals and the anus. Mula bandha is associated with the first two chakras: *muladhara chakra* and *svadisthana chakra*.

Uddiyana banda: stomach lock. Here you pull the navel in towards the spine to increase core strength. *Uddiyana banda* in asana training includes pulling in the navel to maintain a good core stability, while in pranayama it is used in a similar but deeper manner. Uddiyana bandha is linked to the third and fourth chakras: manipura chakra and anahata chakra.

Jalandhara bandha: throat lock. This more difficult exercise requires flexibility in the neck and back. This is automatically engaged in asanas such as *Halasana* (the Plow) and *Parvatasana* (Mountain pose). It is also used in more challenging breathing exercises. *Jalandhara bandha* is achieved by drawing in the chin against the throat so that the back is stretched and the neck muscles lengthen and relax. Stay stable in the pelvis and belly. You should only integrate jalandhara bandha in your training under the supervision of a qualified yoga teacher. Jalandhara bandha is associated with the fifth and sixth chakras, vishuddha chakra and ajna chakra.

Maha bandha is a combination of all three bandhas.

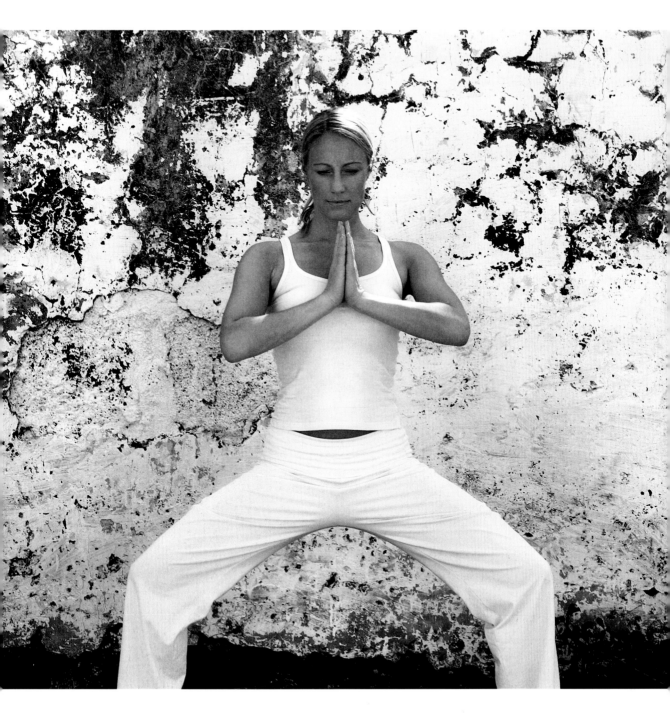

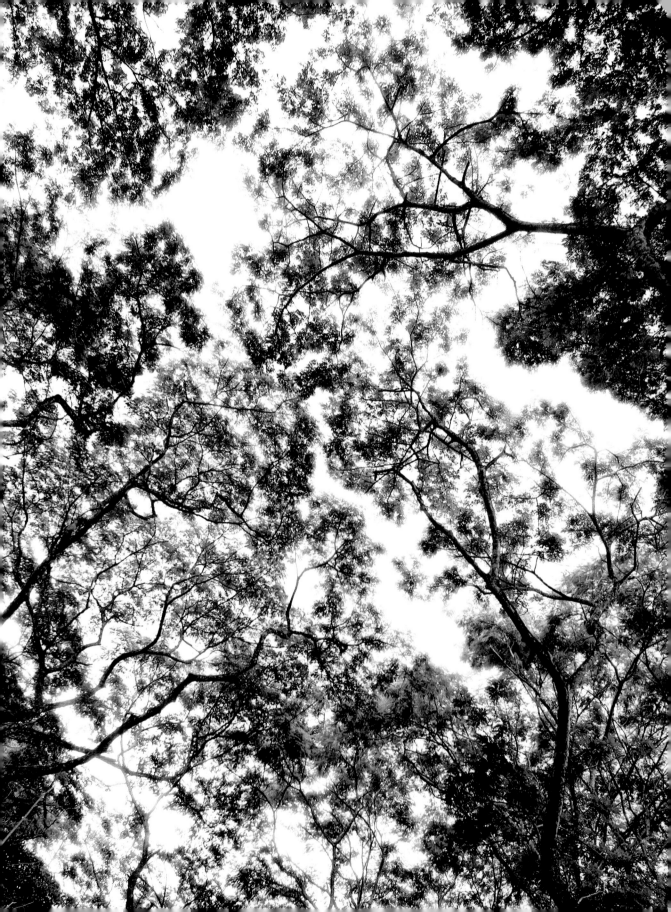

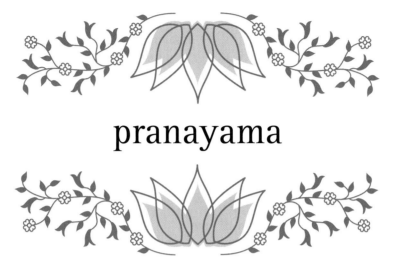

pranayama

We follow the breath to channel our mind's unbalanced behavior.
—Sri O.P. Tiwari

Pranayama is often described as breath control. Although correct in one sense, looking at the many practices pranayama entails shows that this isn't an satisfactory definition. The word pranayama consists of two root words from Sanskrit; prana and yama. Prana means vital energy or life force. Prana is the life-giving energy existing in all living things: plants, animals, and human beings. It is subtler than oxygen and air, although they are close relatives. Yama means control and includes some type of discipline. Originally it was not yama that combined with prana in pranayama, but rather ayama, which has a much deeper significance than yama. Ayama means extension or expansion. Therefore, you could say that a more accurate definition of pranayama would be an extension or expansion of the life force. This extension expresses itself in practice between inhalation and exhalation, so the control of energy happens in the pause between the two. This is more than just exchange of gases in the air sacs of the lungs.

In pranayama you use the breath to influence the prana in the body, as well as to increase prana both inside and out, letting it work as a stimulant to cleanse, regulate, and activate the nadis. In this way, mental and physical stability is achieved.

Pranayama exercises use, train, and strengthen the body's breathing apparatus, but it is more than the exchange of oxygen and carbon dioxide gases. Breath effects energy in the body, the mind, and the soul. Through conscious breathing in tune with nature, breathing as we were meant to, we can strengthen our instrument, the body, so that the mind can have a safer and more secure place to develop.

Yogic exercises force the mind to concentrate, as well as increase blood circulation. Yogic masters maintain that we are born with a fixed quantity of breath. They mean that if we train ourselves to deepen the breath and lengthen the breath, we can live longer. Yogic tradition has always pointed to the importance of and reasons for reflecting on and controlling the breath. It is the breath that is the core of yoga practice—without it we cannot call it Yoga.

Four aspects of a breath

Pranayama divides the breath into four parts, all of which should be respected and paid attention to separately. These are:

1. *Pooraka* (inhalation).

2. *Rechaka* (exhalation).

3. *Antar Kumbhaka* (holding in the inhalation), a pause with oxygen in the lungs. This stabilizes the nervous system, digestion, and the breath.

4. *Bahir Kumbhaka* (holding after exhalation), a pause with carbon dioxide in the lungs. This calms the brain and the nervous system.

These four steps cleanse, settle, and activate the nadis, the body's energy channels. To correctly practice pranayama, the right preconditions, training, and perseverance are needed.

In yoga we concentrate on breathing more effectively by using the diaphragm, keeping the mouth closed, and inhaling and exhaling through the nose (unless you get specific instructions to do otherwise). This is to hold heat in the body and release toxins. Keeping the mouth closed creates a natural counterweight (like using weights in strength training) for the breathing muscles to work with.

Learning the art of breathing correctly is absolutely necessary for good health and increased well-being. When you breathe correctly, you increase lung capacity, which means the blood gets more oxygen, which in turn gives new energy to our inner organs and cleanses them. Conscious and correct breathing works as a calming device for our nervous system: the deeper the breath, the calmer the mind.

Breath, health, and pranayama

Breathing is the most important body process precisely because it affects the activity of every single cell and because it is intimately linked to how the brain and the nervous system perform.

A breath is a complicated process that involves three distinct stages. The first stage occurs between the inhale and the exhale. The oxygen is taken into the upper respiratory passages, through the membranes of the lungs, and then into the bloodstream. The oxygen passes from the air sacs of the lungs into the blood, and through exhalation carbon dioxide (a waste product from metabolism) passes out and is removed from the body. The next step involves oxygen crossing the membranes of the red blood cells to further work through to the body's different cells. In the next and last stage, the cells use the oxygen to build up new cells.

A breath consists of two activities, inhalation and exhalation. Inhalation is a controlled muscular effort. The working muscles are located between the ribs, against the ribs, and in the diaphragm. The diaphragm is used for inhalation. Diaphragmatic breathing requires training to increase the diaphragm's work and to reduce the effort of the chest's expansion. Here we focus on getting the diaphragm to function optimally to make full lung capacity possible. This allows an effective cleansing of wastes and toxins, increased blood circulation, strengthening of the heart, and stimulation of the liver, intestines, and internal organs.

The goal is to lengthen and balance the inhale and the exhale. The reason we do this is to restore control of the breath and become able to steer it. Deep breathing is very calming and can be used any time, especially in Shavasana, Corpse pose.

With correct inhalation, a type of inner massage is supplied to the organs of the stomach. The diaphragm moves down, becomes flattened, and massages the liver when blood is supplied to it, then squeezes it out during exhalation. When we exhale, the crossing abdominal muscles and inner rib muscles are activated, and air that otherwise stays in the lungs is pressed out.

In yoga it is recommended to always exhale with a closed mouth and through the nose. This is to maintain the warmth generated by increased blood circulation, something that improves breathing all by itself, which in turn presses out wastes and toxins from the body.

Pranayama exercise

It is very important to have respect for pranayama and its power. It is also important to follow instructions exactly, as imprecise technique can affect the results to a much greater extent than breath control during asana practice can.

The techniques that you can begin trying on your own (although I strongly recommend that you learn them from a experienced pranayama yoga teacher) are below. Other more challenging exercises I have avoided here, as they require special guidance from a qualified teacher.

Things to think about

The first step is to watch your own breathing and discover your personal breathing style. To become conscious of breath helps the breathing rhythm fall to a more relaxed and balanced level. Start by sitting in a classic breathing position, such as *Padmasana* (see page 43). Scan your own current breathing pattern and reflect on the quality of your breath. Concentrate on achieving inhalations that match the exhalations in length. This strengthens the lungs and balances the nervous system and the pranic system of the body.

If you have never practiced cleansing pranayama, some symptoms can emerge along with the training. You may start to feel itchy, ticklish inside your head, unusually cold or hot, light or heavy. These effects are temporary and generally disappear quickly. The reason they arise is that the liver and the kidneys are pushing out the body's wastes and toxins. If they remain, consult your doctor and an experienced pranayama yoga teacher.

Avoid practicing pranayama exercises when you are sick, have a fever, or are mentally unbalanced.

Ujjayi Bandha Pranayama, *Nadi Shodhana*, *Sheetali*, and *Bhramari* should be practiced before or after asanas, in a sitting position.

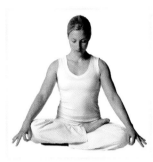

Ujjayi Pranayama: winning breath

The activating breath: a fantastic technique for strengthening the diaphragm, increasing blood circulation, and calming the mind. This type of breath is advised for use in asana training, or even as a pure pranayama technique. In combination with asana training it is a complete tool to even out imbalances, find stamina and strength, come into balance, increase flexibility and agility, and cleanse the body.

1. Sit in Padmasana. Start by focusing on the exhale. Exhale with the mouth closed and concentrate on letting the lower part of the chest settle down and in toward the spine. This causes all the air to be pressed out from the lungs. Hold for a little while. Relax the hold and you'll notice that you automatically inhale.

2. Next, when you exhale, whisper an "ahhh" or an "uuu" sound with an open mouth. Feel the soft vibration deep within the throat. Then whisper "ahhh" or "uuu" on the inhale.

3. Now breathe in the same way but with a closed mouth. Your inhalation will make a laboring sound, while the exhalation will come to have more of a hissing sound. Think about "drawing up" the inhalation from the hips up the spine and through the chest, and then let the exhale happen slowly, as if you are holding it in just a bit. If you start to cough or feel queasy while you are doing the Ujjayi breath, you are trying too hard. Think of soft, long breaths with relaxed shoulders and open chest. Try to expand the chest through the breastbone.

Ujjayi Bandha Pranayama: the deep breath

Diaphragmatic, deep breathing: this pranayama technique is a very good way to develop respiratory stamina, pelvic floor strength, and mental focus.

1. Sit in Padmasana. Close your eyes and find your Ujjayi breath. Press the tongue lightly against the roof of the mouth. When you have found the breath you may proceed.

2. Let the next exhalation completely empty the lungs. Hold the breath.

3. Integrate the *mula bandha*, breathing in at the same time that you slowly count to five (in your head).

4. Hold the breath (*antar kumbhaka*) and count silently to two. Continue to hold mula bandha.

5. Then add *Uddiyana bandha* during the exhalation at the same time that you slowly count to five. When you continue the exhalation, release the root lock gradually and transition to letting the abdominal lock become more active. (Imagine it as the same pull when you change gears when driving a car.)

6. Hold the breath (*bahir kumbhaka*) and release all the holds. Count slowly to two.

7. Repeat, for a total of 10 times.

8. Lay in Shavasana, Corpse pose, and rest for one minute.

This breathing practice calms the nervous system and the mind and has a balancing effect on the psyche and body. Ujjayi can be done sitting, lying, or standing. Try not to tighten the face or jaw when you are working with Ujjayi beathing (it is quite common to do this when a breathing technique has many different components).

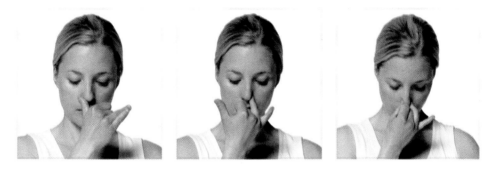

Nadi Shodhana: Cleansing the nerve channels

This is an alternative breath through the nostrils. It is one of the oldest and most well-known pranayama techniques. There are many variations of the technique, depending on the practitioner's readiness as well as the goal. This technique is extremely effective in increasing vitality in the nervous system and the organs and lowering stress levels and physical anxiety. It also brings focus, calm, and clarity.

1. Sit in a comfortable position with a straight back, palms facing upward on the knees. Let the index finger and the thumb meet (*Chin Mudra*). Then form the right hand into Hridaya Mudra. Place the right thumb and the ring finger on either side of the nostrils in Nasagra Mudra. Relax the other fingers. ALWAYS start with inhalation on the left side.

2. Exhale completely and close the right nostril with the right thumb, holding the breath at the same time that you count to four.

3. Then inhale gently through the left nostril

4. Hold the breath and close both nostrils with the ring finger and the thumb, and count to two.

5. Release the thumb and exhale slowly via the right nostril to the count of four.

6. Hold the breath for a count of two.

7. Inhale via the right nostril.

8. Hold the breath for a count of two, closing both nostrils.

9. Release the ring finger and exhale through the left nostril.

10. That was one round. The rhythm is: left, close, out the right, in the right, close, out the left, and so on. Then lie in Shavasana and rest for one minute.

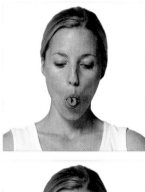

Sheetali (sitali): the cooling breath

Sheetali comes from the word sheet, which means cool. Sheetal means "that which is calm, soft, and without distractions." Sheetali has a calming effect on the body, mind, and emotions, promotes digestion, and neutralizes gas and sourness in the intestines. It creates calming energy through the musculature so you can more easily relax. This technique is excellent to practice after asanas or other yogic practices that create heat in the body.

1. Sit relaxed with a straight back. Rest the palms on the knees in *Chin* or *Jnana mudra*. Close the eyes and relax.
2. Stick out your tongue as far as you can without straining and make it into a tube. Slowly breathe in through the "tube."
3. Close the mouth and exhale (ujjayi). Your breath should sound like a swift wind.
4. Repeat 10 times.
5. Don't force it. Slow and smooth. Release the jaw.
6. Lay in *Shavasana* and rest for one minute.

Some people cannot form a tube with their tongue as described above. If you are one that cannot, then practice a similar pranayama technique called *Sitkari* (which means hissing in Sanskrit). Instead of rolling the tongue sideways you press the tip of the tongue backwards against the upper teeth. Follow the same procedure above.

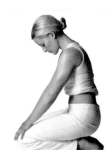

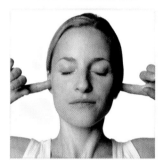

Bhramari: buzzing bee breath

Bhramari means bee; this breathing technique is named after the sound bees make in flight. This method is effective in reducing stress and muscle tension in the neck, back, and face. Making the bee noise creates a vibration in the sinus cavity and throat, which loosens up excess mucus. It can result in the need to spit or blow your nose. Bhramari shouldn't be practiced lying down, and those that suffer from acute ear infections should avoid this exercise completely until an infection has cleared up.

1. Sit in relaxed position with a straight spine, hands on the knees. Close your eyes and relax throughout the body.

2. Stretch your chest and your throat and feel how the spine lengthens. Avoid rounding the back. Keep the mouth closed, but relax the jaw so that you can feel the vibration in the mouth, throat, and sinuses.

3. Stop your ears with your index fingers. Relax the shoulders. Focus in on the crown of the head, where Ajna chakra is located, and keep the body still. Inhale slowly and deeply.

4. Exhale slowly and steadily while humming "mmm" in a low but audible tone. The humming shouldn't be forced, but it should be more than a whisper. If you feel the area around the forehead vibrating, you are doing it right. At the end of the exhale, stop humming, take a new inhale, and repeat 5-10 times. Then rest in Shavasana for one minute.

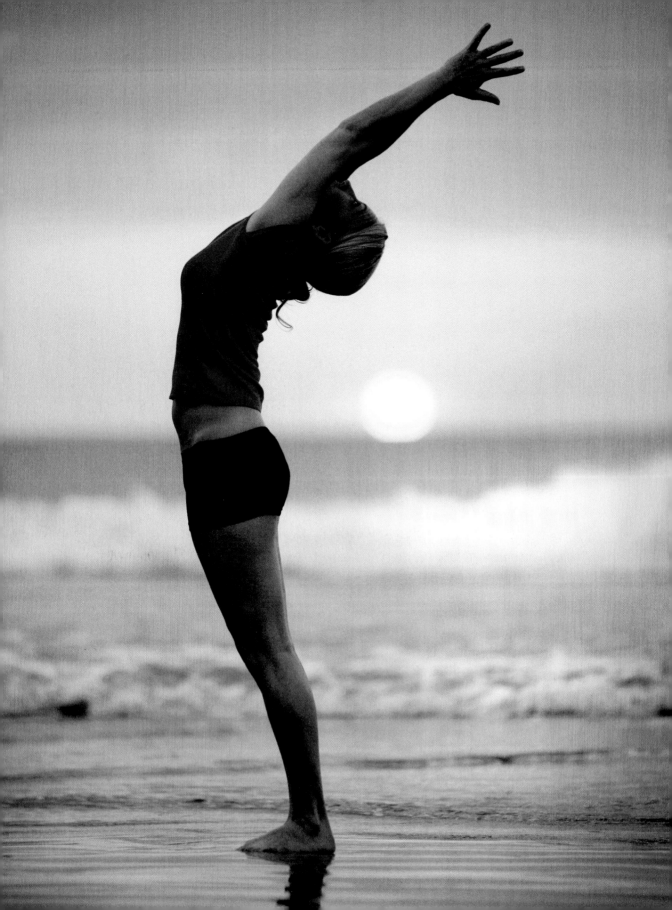

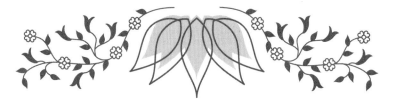

surya and chandra

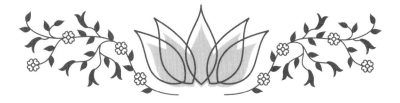

The yogi completely filled with wisdom and insight, who stands with quiet mind unmoved
by the sight of clod of earth, stone or gold—that would be called an anchored being.
—Bhagavad Gita 6.7

Sun salutations and moon salutations are fundamental in Hatha Yoga. It is common to start your practice with sun/moon salutations after a short period of focusing on the breath. These salutations are a good foundation for the rest of training and contribute to warming the body and bringing focus to the mind. Each sun and moon salutation is a complete exercise set that can be seen as a warm-up for the muscles and joints as well as the mind and soul.

Surya Namaskara: Sun salutation

Surya, sun in Sanskrit, was an ancient Indian symbol for the clear insight people hoped to develop within themselves. Sun salutations include three parts: form, energy, and rhythm. The twelve positions in sun salutations create the form. These asanas generate prana through the body. The way they are done, in concert with the breath, gives them a steady rhythm that symbolizes the twenty-four hours of the day, the twelve signs of the zodiac (how the sun travels around the earth in a year), and the body's biorhythm. When form meets rhythm, energy is created, not only for the present moment but also stretching into the future. Sun salutations are ideal to practice before other asanas.

The twelve positions should be done one time on each leg to balance the two sides of the body—in other words, an entire sun salutation is twenty-four positions. Positions 1 though 12 are a half-round, and the other half repeats, except for that in position 4 (which would be the sixteenth position), *Ashwa Sanchalanasana*, you step back with the left foot, and in position 9 (or position 21), *Ashwa Sanchalanasana*, you step forward with the left foot. After a complete sun salutation, twenty-four positions, take four deep breaths before you do one more complete (twenty-four positions) round.

Avoid these exercises if you have untreated high blood pressure, coronary artery disease, or have had a stroke, and avoid them if you have any type of infection. Consult your doctor or an experienced yoga teacher if you are at all unsure.

Chandra Namaskara: Moon salutation

Chandra means moon in Sanskrit. The moon is a symbol for humanity's inner wisdom and mental strength: in other words, inner security, harmony, higher consciousness, and increased knowledge. According to yogic tradition, practicing moon salutations causes the body and the nervous system to experience increased nourishment and energy. The moon's sustaining influence also serves to balance the immune system. Moon salutations are said to influence creativity in the body, mind, and soul.

The fourteen positions in moon salutations symbolize the different phases of the moon as it circles around the earth. Do moon salutations in the evening, especially when the moon is out. You should be well-versed in sun salutations before beginning moon salutations, since all the positions except for one are the same as in the sun salutations. The added position, *Ardha Chandrasana*, gives increased balance and concentration. To get here, inhale and lift the upper body and arms and let the palms meet, then exhale into parvatasana.

An entire moon salutation should, like an entire sun salutation, be done once on each leg, for a total of twenty-eight positions. In the second half you do the same as in the first half, except that in position 4 (18), *Ashwa Sanchalasana*, lunge pose, take a step back with the right foot, and in position 10 (24), *Ashwa Sanchalasana*, take a step forward with the right foot.

After an entire round, take four deep breaths before you attempt another full round. It is common to do four complete rounds, but how many times you do it depends on your goal. For increased balanced breath you should do three to seven rounds at an easy pace. To increase your physical balance beyond that, do three to twelve rounds with a bit more power.

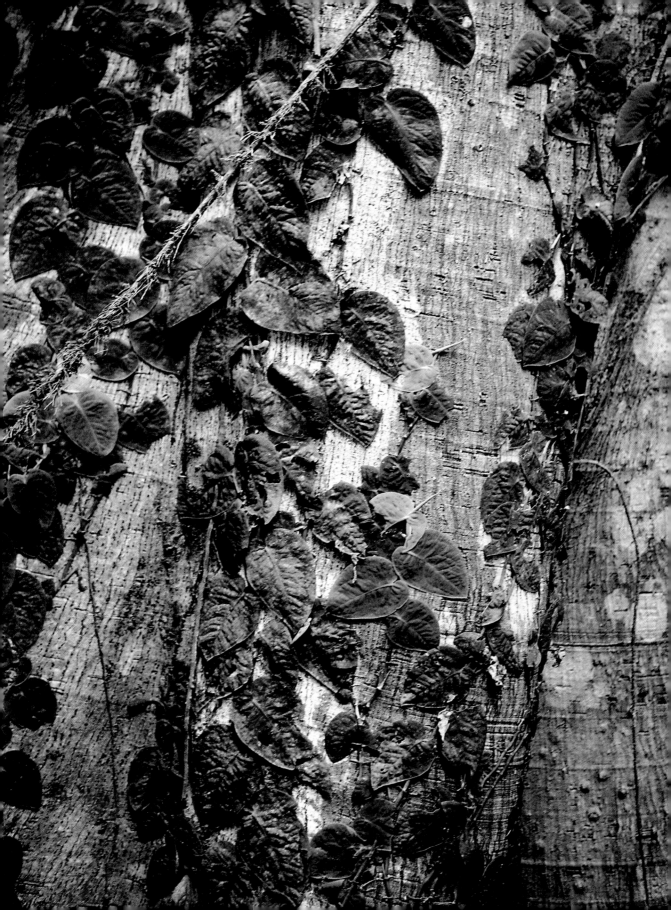

Surya namaskara: Sun salutation

On pages 56-62 each of the individual poses is described in more detail.

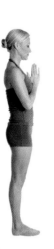

1. *Pranamasana*

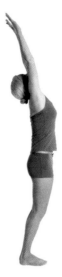

2. *Hasta Uttanasana*

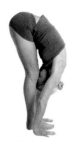

3. *Padahastasana*

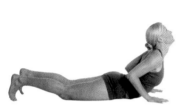

7. *Bhujangasana*

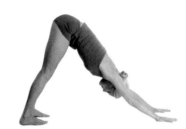

8. *Parvatasana*

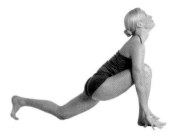

9. *Ashwa Sanchalanasana*

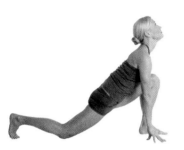

4. Ashwa Sanchalanasana

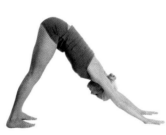

5. Parvatasana

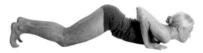

6. Ashtanga Namaskara

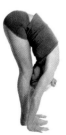

10. Padahastasana

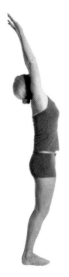

11. Hasta Uttanasana

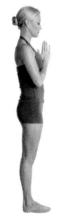

12. Pranamasana

Chandra namaskara: Moon salutation

On pages 56-63 each of the individual poses is described in more detail.

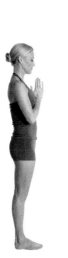
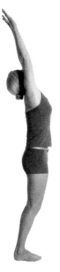
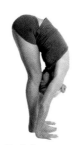
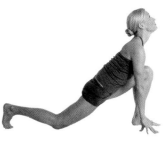

1. Pranamasana   2. Hasta Uttanasana   3. Padahastasana   4. Ashwa Sanchalanasana

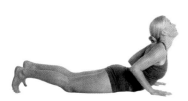
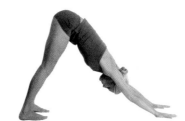
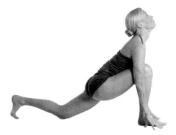

8. Bhujangasana   9. Parvatasana   10. Ashwa Sanchalanasana

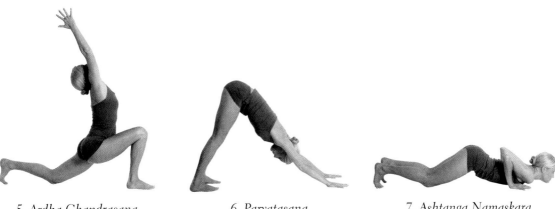

5. Ardha Chandrasana

6. Parvatasana

7. Ashtanga Namaskara

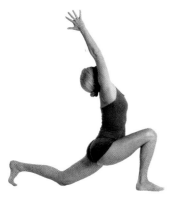

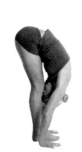

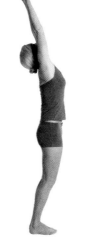

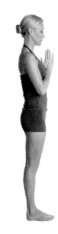

11. Ardha Chandrasana

12. Padahastasana

13. Hasta Uttanasana

14. Pranamasana

Pranamasana: Prayer pose

Begins and ends both sun and moon salutations, is followed by Hasta Uttanasana.

From *Tadasana* (see page 76)
Bend the elbows slowly and bring the hands together in front of the chest in *Anjali mudra*. Relax and breathe calmly and deeply.

Drishti: Close the eyes or look down the tip of the nose
Bandhas: *Mula, Uddiyana, Jalandhara bandha*

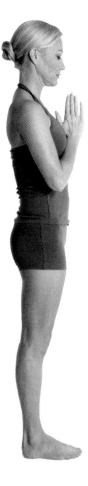

This position helps create calm and concentration for the following movements. Pranamasana is followed by Hasta Uttanasana. This position should both start and end sun and moon salutations. When you finish a sequence, return to Pranamasana from Hasta Uttanasana.

Hasta Uttanasana: Raised hands pose

Preceded by Pranamasana or Padahastasana and followed by Padahastasana or Pranamasana.

As you finish Pranamasana, you begin the salutation sequence: lower your arms to your sides. Imagine grabbing the inhale from behind you as you bend the knees, roll the hips inward to be in line with the trunk, inhale and lift the chest and arms up over the head. Relax the shoulders. You will return here from Padahastasana again in the sequence: at that point move up slowly so that your arms are raised and in position.

Drishti: at your thumbs
Bandhas: *Mula banda*

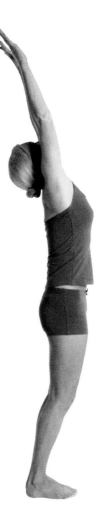

This position improves digestion. It trains arm and shoulder muscles, strengthens spinal nerves, opens the lungs, and increases circulation, especially in the front of the body.

Padahastasana: Hands-to-feet forward bend

Preceded in the lead-in to both sun and moon salutation by Hasta Uttanasana and followed by Ashwa Sanchalansana. At the end of the sun salutation, Padahastasana is preceded by Ashwa Sanchalansana, and at the end of the moon salutation this position is preceded by Ardha Chandrasana.

From Hasta Uttanasana: Follow the thumbs with your eyes and stretch the body. On the exhale: follow the thumbs as you bend carefully forward from the hips, keeping a straight back and slightly bent knees. Place the palms on either side of the foot. Bend your knees if you can't come all the way down with the hands. At the end of the sun salutation you come from Ashwa Sanchalanasana, or Ardha Chandrasana at the end of the moon salutation, and follow the thumbs down into the position.

Drishti: Follow thumbs down to the knees, then the navel
Bandhas: *Uddiyana bandha*

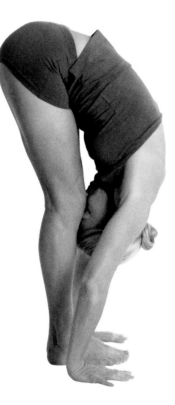

This position stimulates digestion, strengthens the spinal column and spinal nerves, increases blood circulation in the hips, loins, and pelvis, and relieves constipation.

Ashwa Sanchalanasana: Low lunge

Preceded in the introduction of both sun and moon salutations by Padahastasana, before Parvatanasana. In the introduction of the sun salutation, this position is followed by Parvatasana, after Padahastasana. In both the beginning and the end of the moon salutation, it is followed by Ardha Chandrasana.

From Padahastasana: During the inhale, take a lunge back with the right foot, keep the gaze looking up past the nose, and lift the chest. Roll the shoulders back and place the fingertips on the floor. Relax the shoulders, the throat, the jaw, and the face. You will return to this position at the end of the salutation from Parvatanasana, after which you will step forward with the right leg.

Drishti: Follow the gaze past the nose, looking up towards the sky
Bandhas: *Mula* and *Uddiyana bandha*

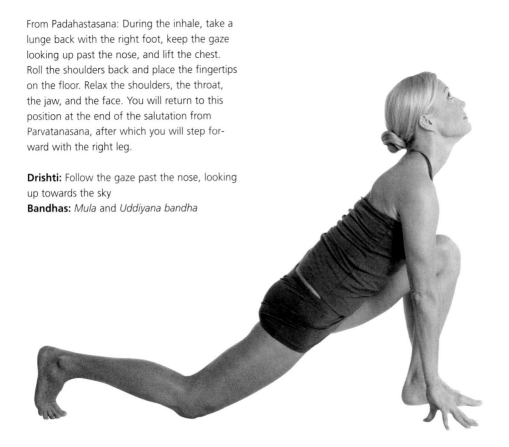

This position massages the inner organs and strengthens them, strengthens the leg muscles, and balances the nerve system. Ashwa Sanchalanasana is followed in the sun salutation by Parvatasana (see the following page) and in the moon salutation by Ardha Chandrasana (see page 63).

Parvatanasana: Mountain-top pose

Preceeded in the introduction of the sun salutation by Ashwa Sanchalanasana, in the introduction of the moon salutation by Ardha Chandrasana. At the end of both the sun and the moon salutation it proceeds Bhujangasana. In the beginning of both the sun and moon salutation it is followed by Ashtanga Namaskara; in the end it is followed by Ashwa Sanchalanasana.

You move into this pose from Ashwa Sanchalanasana at the beginning of the sun salutation and Ardha Chandrasana at the beginning of the moon salutation.

1. From all fours, your hands should be directly under your shoulders and your knees directly under your hips. Spread out your fingers and push down through the palms and the soles of the feet.

2. Exhale, lifting the knees. At first keep the knees bent and the heels lifted. Relax the soles of the feet. Lift the tailbone.

3. Push the seat bones up to the sky at the same time that you inhale. Relax the head between the arms.

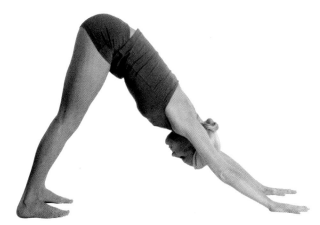

4. Inhale and pull the navel in toward the spine. Exhale and engage the front of the thighs, push down through the big toes without lifting the heels. Stretch out gently through the knees and the back.

5. Press the shoulder blades down toward the back of the chest; imagine that you are moving the floor with the hands and stretch out the shoulder blades without folding the shoulders in toward each other.

At the end of the sequence you come to this pose from Bhujangasana.

Drishti: Looking to the legs for beginners, gazing in toward the navel for more advanced practitioners
Bandhas: *Mula* and *Uddiyana bandha*

This position is also called *Adho Mukha Svanasana* (Downward facing dog). It calms the brain and relieves stress and depression, gives the body energy, stretches the shoulders, the back of the thighs, calves, wrists, and hands, and strengthens arms and legs. Ask your teacher for alternative hand positions if you suffer from numbness in the hands. Avoid this position if you have diarrhea.

Ashtanga Namaskara: Eight-limbed salute

This is preceded by Parvatasana and followed by Bhujangasana in both the sun and moon salutation.

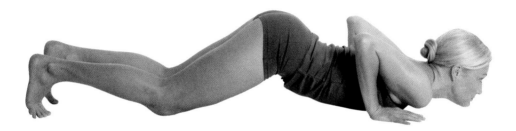

You get here from Parvatasana: Hold the breath, sink the knees, chest, and chin down into the mat. The hips, seat, and belly are up in the air.

Drishti: Third eye, between the eyebrows
Bandhas: *Uddiyana bandha*

This position strengthens arm and leg muscles, develops the chest, and trains the area between the shoulder blades.

Bhujangasana: Cobra

This is preceded by Ashtanga Namaskara and followed by Parvatasana.

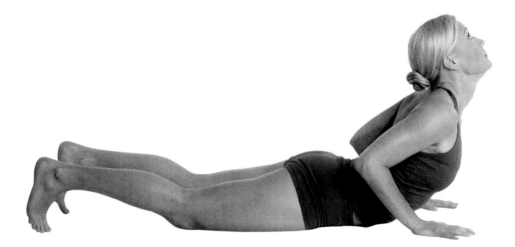

Come to this position from Ashtanga Namaskara: Lower the hips, thighs, and lower belly to the floor. While inhaling, look past the tip of the nose toward the sky, lifting the chest, and curve the back, drawing the shoulder blades together and down toward the lower back.

Keep the arms bent. Spread the fingers and keep the pelvic floor, navel, palms, and fingers stable.

Drishti: Looking up toward the sky
Bandhas: *Mula* and *Uddiyana bandha*

This position strengthens and stabilizes the lower back, improves the circulation in the back muscles, and strengthens the spinal nerves. In addition, the reproductive organs are strengthened, the liver, kidneys, adrenal glands, and digestive organs are improved, and the risk of constipation lessened.

Ardha Chandrasana: Half-moon pose

This position only appears in moon salutation and is preceded by Ashwa Sanchalasana. The pose is followed at the start of the sequence by Parvatasana and at the end by Padahastasana.

Come to this pose from Ashwa Sanchalanasana. Completely exhale. On your next inhale, lift the hips, chest, eyes, chin, and arms up toward the sky and let the hands meet over the head. Keep the arms stretched, and relax in the shoulders. Feel the muscular support from the legs, navel, and pelvic floor.

The movement should resemble a half-moon: think about the body creating this by forming a soft bow from the finger tips to the toes. This position develops physical and psychic balance and is a fantastic whole-body stretch.

Drishti: Looking up toward the sky.
Bandhas: *Mula* and *Uddiyana bandha*

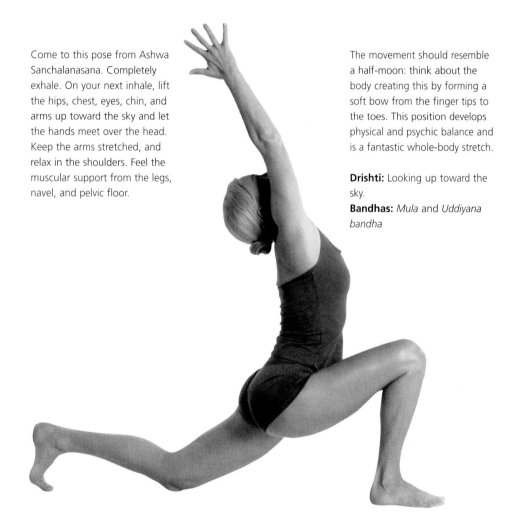

Ardha Chandrasana is only included in moon salutations. In the beginning of the sequence the left leg should be forward, and at the end the right leg should be forward.

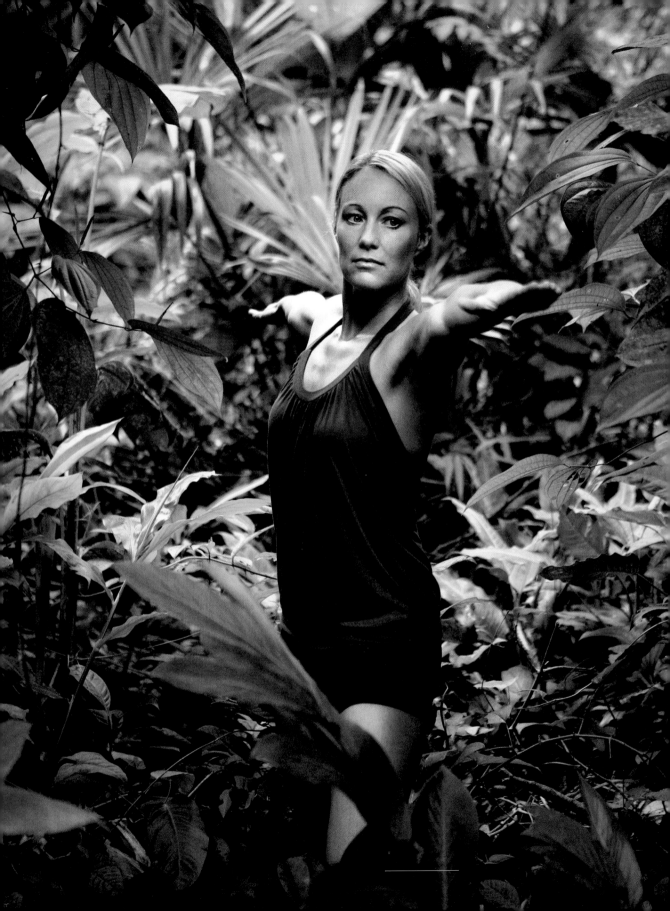

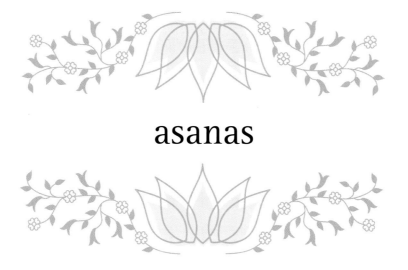

asanas

You are no older than the age of your spine. — Yogic saying

One of the key elements in asana practice is to sit and stand with good posture; thus, many of the exercises are meant to strengthen the abdominal muscles and lower back so that you can maintain a straight spine. Regardless of whether you are standing, sitting, or kneeling, you should imagine a string drawing up the spine.

Yoga asanas are often seen as a form of exercise and physical training. They are not. Asanas are a technique for placing the body in different positions in order to increase consciousness, relaxation, strength, and concentration. Asana training in Hatha Yoga is chiefly concerned with breath-controlled body positioning using bandhas, mudras, and drishti. Even if yoga asanas are not simply a physical exercise program, they do work together with other forms of physical training. If you don't train and strengthen the body, the muscles deteriorate, the skeletal frame is weakened, oxygen intake is reduced, insulin sensitivity can increase, and physical fitness is drastically reduced. There are many similarities between yoga asanas and other forms of fitness, but just as many differences.

Asanas are all different symbols for the various challenges we encounter in life. How you experience a pose is how you perceive yourself in life, in the same type of challenge. Asanas make you aware of your strong and weak sides, and by training both dimensions they come to work more in harmony with each other. Often it is the positions you like least that you need the most. The objective in asanas is to feel peaceful and strong in the pose. If the pose feels challenging you will need to do it again and again, or perhaps simplify it until it feels that you can achieve it and, over time, improve upon it. It is very important to take this idea to heart, because we humans are often in a hurry and tend to rush ahead as quickly as possible. This creates a huge risk for injury and can drain our energy. Everything has its own time. Listen to your yoga teacher if he or she wants you to hold back. They might know from experience that you can injure yourself or aren't quite ready to advance, and have only your own well-being in mind.

When you take part in a yoga class your teacher will take you through a series of poses that always include asanas from those described below. Each pose has its counterpose. If you've, for example, just bent forward, you'll probably follow with a back bend. This is to keep balance in the musculature and joints as well as in the spine.

Hatha Yoga divides asanas into different groupings. This is the classical division of poses: standing poses, forward bends, back bends, arm or toe balancing poses, sitting positions, twists, inversions, and resting poses.

Some asanas are used for several purposes and are included in more than one of the groups. It all depends on which poses come before and after, what is its current purpose, what breathing goes along with it (which technique, the length of the breath, the focus, etc.). In other words, how, when, and what the pose is useful for. The most important things to remember in asanas are posture, gaze, and breath. Posture is a requirement for the other two to work, so try to put your body into the movement in the right way instead of going for a perfect appearance. Work with your body, not against it. With many of the poses described in this chapter you'll find information about which effect you should be aiming for. These effects are achieved only after you have done the complete set of poses and are doing yoga regularly.

Advice and help on practicing asanas

1. Strive for correct placement of feet and hands and drishti, and be aware of how you hold your body through the different asanas, where your muscular/mental support comes from (bandhas, breath focus), the quality of the breath, etc.

2. Try to accept yourself instead of judging yourself in the pose. Don't compare yourself to others or to yourself on a different day. Try to see your body as new each time you come onto the mat.

3. Relax your face when you do exercises. Always try to keep your focus on the breath. If your thoughts take hold of you or you lose focus, take a pause in *Balasana*, Child's pose, to find the breath once more.

4. Be consistent with the relaxing poses after the more physically challenging poses. *Always* end with Shavasana, Corpse pose, for at least 7-10 minutes, after the asana practice.

5. Shower before training and scrub the skin to remove dirt and dead skin cells; wash your feet and clip your nails.

6. Relieve your bladder and your bowels if possible. Many positions in combination with each other can stimulate the bowels. Advanced positions require empty bowels. Always wear clean, loose clothing to practice.

7. Asanas should be done on an empty stomach (not hungry). This is due to the fact that it facilitates mental focus, power, and concentration on breathing. It is also best to hydrate before and after practice rather than during.

8. Avoid doing asanas after you've spent a long time in the sun, as it will tend to be tiring rather than rejuvenating.

9. Avoid asanas and some pranayama techniques during the first three days of menstruation. Even if you don't ever feel discomfort when working out during your period, take it easy, especially in the up and down positions.

10. If you are pregnant I recommend a yoga class especially for pregnant women. Even if you are an experienced practitioner you should take it easy and consult with your yoga teacher. After your pregnancy, you should wait about a month before starting up asana practice. When you do start, listen to your body. Consult with your midwife and yoga teacher if you feel unsure.

11. Listen to your own physical requirements and adjust the yoga to fit with them.

12. If you are in any way insecure or unsure, consult your doctor or yoga teacher before you start asanas or pranayama.

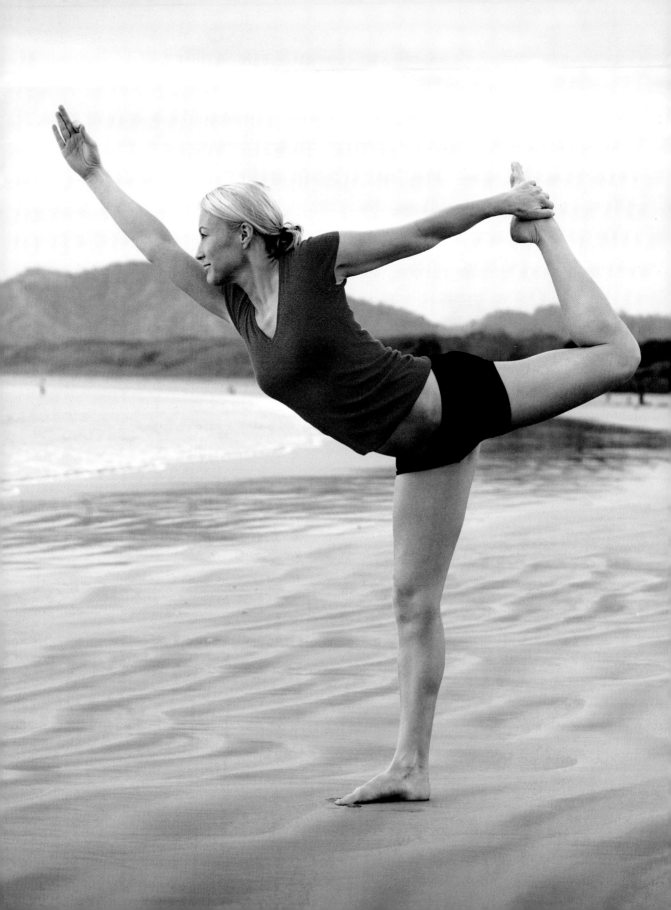

Focus on the breath during asanas

For many, working out lets them put aside thoughts of work, duties, and responsibilities and increases their stamina for other things. You feel more alive and stronger. But even so the stress might remain, manifesting itself as bad digestion, bad skin, headaches, and difficulty relaxing. Inner calm and happiness might remain elusive.

When the breath is stronger and we achieve increased focus on breath, our body awareness also increases. The feeling of the right body position in different asanas gives increased balance, and our posture in the movement is improved, giving us more ability to further develop the yoga pose. By developing a more powerful, stronger breath, the poses are also easier, the muscles are warmer and softer, and you will feel that your mind calms down and harmony is achieved. All the different parts of you begin to work together on the same frequency, and the beginning of well-being starts to manifest itself. You feel strong, focused and calm; other thoughts don't come in to bother you during practice. Your body is happy because you have filled it with energy and it gives you acknowledgement in the form of endorphins.

Some of the most common asanas

The various poses or positions of yoga have developed over hundreds of years. The names of the poses have different sources depending on how they have developed. Some of the names describe the shape or form the body takes while doing the pose, others are taken from nature. Some have even gotten their name from the masters of the form. Then there are names that remind us why do a certain pose. Even if the name is decided by tradition, poses can be called different names in different yoga styles or traditions.

In Hatha Yoga we work first and foremost preventatively and then constructively over time to master the basics, without forcing either the body or the mind. Only then can we be ready to develop the poses further. In any case, it isn't recommended to go too far with one pose if the pose leading up to it or following immediately after can't be mastered. All asanas have a relationship to the others. This is to create balance both in the musculature and the nervous system. Each position has a counterposition; thus the order in which the positions are done during a class is important.

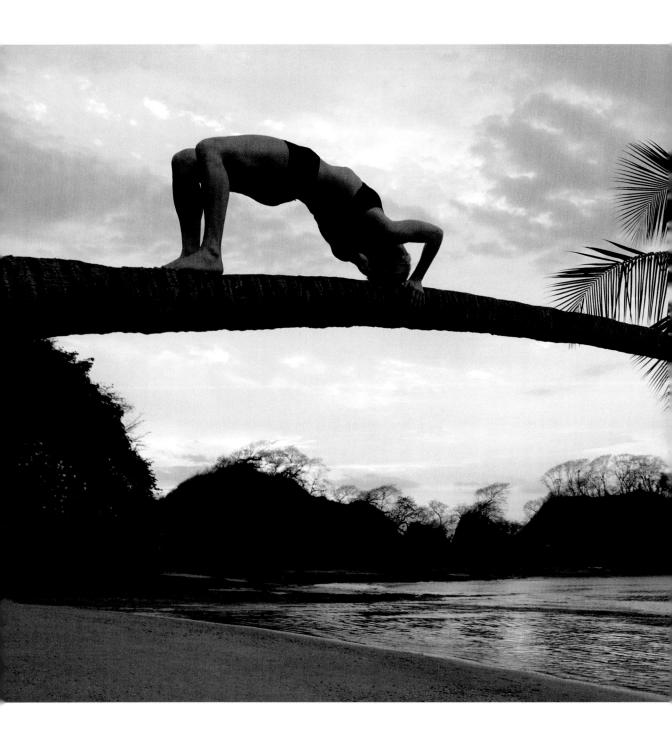

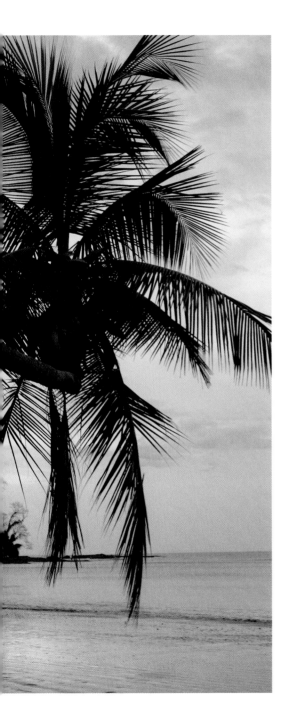

In each asana think about the following to maintain good posture:

- Foot/hand placement
- Point of concentration for the gaze, drishti
- Breath (increasing blood circulation, settling the mind)
- Legs (support for the back)
- Abdomen (bandhas support for hips, back, neck, see page 34)
- Heart, positioning of the chest (to avoid over-working the neck and upper spine)
- Shoulders (keep them relaxed to avoid over-working the neck)
- Chin/jaw (keep relaxed and in line with the spine)

On the following pages you can go over the current best-known and most-practiced basic poses.

Standing poses (pages 76-84)

According to yogic tradition, it is the standing positions that aim to develop strength and power. They teach us perfect posture, self-esteem, balance, presence, and engagement and help us to handle everyday life better. You'll come to see that when you lose your balance it is because you started thinking about something else and lost your focus on the breath or on the gaze. "Where you are on the mat shows you where you are in life," is a classic saying in yoga. Accept, don't judge, just do the work—strive for balance!

Forward bending (pages 85-87)

While back bends work against the power of gravity, we use gravity in forward bends to release tension, stress, and pains in our musculature on both the back side and the front of the body. Forward bends release muscular tension in the back and the back of the legs. These asanas move the spinal column into a position that is called the primary curve, the shape it had in the womb. When you bend the body over the legs (with a stretched spine), each vetebrae in the spine is separated, which stimulates the nerves, increases the circulation around the spine, reduces compression in the vertebral column, and increases the supply of energy to the large nerves of the back.

Be aware that forward bends should be initiated from the hips (the groin), not from the waist. This gives a greater range of movement and creates space for the abdominal muscles to work to keep the back in the right position. Be careful not to force the back into something it is not ready for. Be careful of yourself. Strive for correct technique and deep breathing and let gravity do its job. If you do a forward bend from a sitting position, sit on the area between the pubic bone and the seat bones instead of on the tailbone. Don't forget to use your arms and your hands to help support correct posture.

Backbends (pages 88-90)

Backbends are asanas that turn the body outward to the world. They expand the chest and release the tensions there, both at the front and back, and strengthen the muscles in the back, between the ribs, shoulders, and abdomen.

These poses increase flexibility in the abdominal muscles and strengthens the muscles that control the spinal column, which leads to the relief and prevention of many back problems. If you have or have had problems with the back, I advise you to turn to an experienced yoga teacher and ask for help.

Recent research has show that 90 percent of the most common chronic back problems are due to muscle problems and poor posture. If these imbalances continue for a longer time, the spinal column can change (the vertebrae can be dislocated, the ligaments can be strained, and the discs can give way), which means that imbalances and discomfort will be much worse.

Backbends increase circulation to the back of the body. As with all asanas, it is important to do them correctly and in concert with the breath and posture, so that the correct muscles are working.

Arm/toe balancing poses (pages 91-93)

All balance asanas strengthen the cerebellum, the center in the brain that controls how the body functions in a movement. Many people are uncoordinated in their movements, which leads to their bodies constantly having to compensate for a lack of balance so that they don't fall or bring things down around them. This means the body has to work its hardest, resulting in extra stress for the body. Balancing poses develop a balanced mind and a mature approach to life.

Balancing poses neutralize stress and disturbances in the body and the mind. The yogic approach is to try to hold the poses as long as possible while maintaining conscious breathing and focus. Balancing poses can be difficult in the beginning, but you can quickly improve. It is important to keep a strong gaze and point of concentration and to focus on inhaling and exhaling.

Sitting positions and twists (page 94-102)

These asanas contribute to abdomen and spinal column strength and flexibility. Here we work to move the energy from the chest, and the focus lies on the back and the hips. Many of these positions also increase the movement and strength in the hip joints, knees, thighs, feet, back of the thighs, front of the thighs, and all of the back muscles.

All the sitting positions start from Dandasana. Sit with a straight back on the mat with the legs stretched in front of you. "Rock" back with the seat until you feel that you settle on the seat bones. If it feels difficult, bend the legs. Stretch the toes up, engage the front of the thighs, and press the legs together. Place the hands on either side of the hips, on the mat. Lift the chest and aim your gaze at your toes. Stay here for five long, deep breaths.

Inversions (up and down) (pages 103-106)

Inversions work against gravity and turn the body upside down. They improve overall health, reduce stress, and calm body and mind while increasing self-esteem. They develop mental strength, the ability to concentrate, and the ability to tolerate stress. These asanas increase the blood supply to the brain, which nourishes the nerve cells and helps to drive out toxins from the body. When the body is upside down the breath is automatically calmed, which leads to maximization of the exchange of oxygen and carbon dioxide, something that increases the lung capacity. This group of asanas should be done carefully and correctly in a way that fits the individual. They are incredibly important in yoga training because they bring down the body's tempo in order to allow it to start to relax.

Exercises in which the hips are lifted over the heart are called inversions and should be avoided by:
• Women during the first two to three days of menstruation.
• Pregnant women (if they are not already experienced yogis—always consult with the yoga teacher).
• Those with uncontrolled high blood pressure and or high cholesterol.
• Those suffering from obesity, as well as those who have just undergone an operation on the eyes or plastic surgery. Talk with your doctor first!
• Those that have a "locked" back, either in the upper or lower back. Consult a professional yoga teacher or a chiropractor if you are unsure.

Resting poses (page 107-108)

I can't stress enough the importance of resting poses. Neglecting these in asana training cuts results in half. They should always be part of the ending phase of your daily yoga program and should be returned to anytime that you feel tired. It may seem like they're easy to do half-way, but they are strenuous and really require correct technique to bring a feeling of harmony and energy and release of the tensions in the body. Sometimes we believe that the muscles are relaxed after we have stretched, but the truth is they often remain tense. To rest by sleeping doesn't give exactly the same recovery for the nervous system and the muscles. To rest in relaxation poses is a must for the total effect. Resting poses give the spine a complete energy recharge.

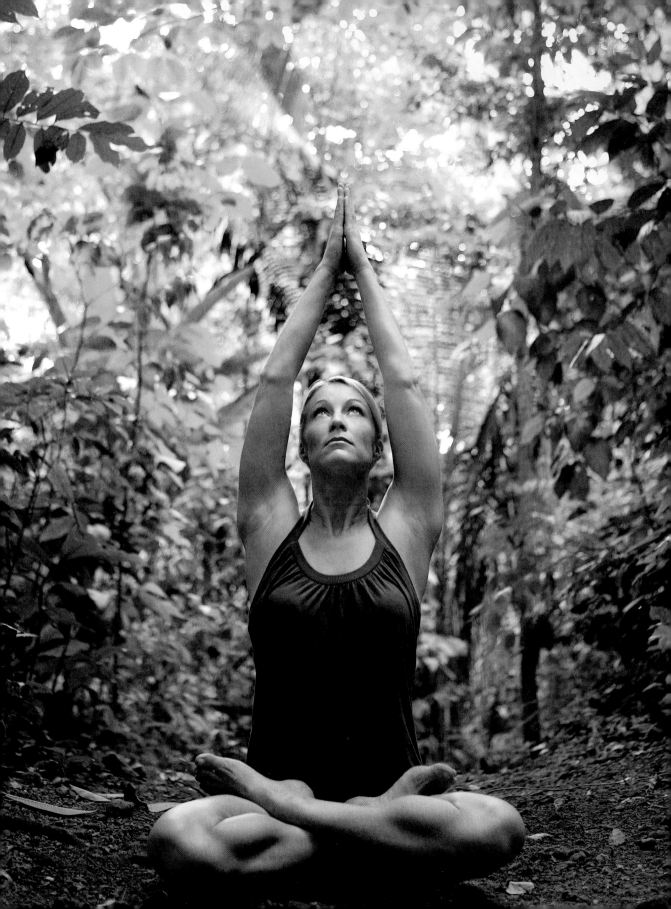

Tadasana: Mountain pose

Tada = mountain

1. Straighten the spine, stand with feet together. Make sure that you are standing on the entire sole of the foot and that the big toes meet, as do the heels. Engage the front of the thighs and try to make the hips line up.

2. Engage both *Mula* and *Uddiyana bandha* to give support to the lower back and to establish abdominal support. Lift the chest so that the back stretches up. Relax the shoulders and roll them back.

Drishti: tip of the nose
Bandhas: *Mula* and *Uddiyana* bandha

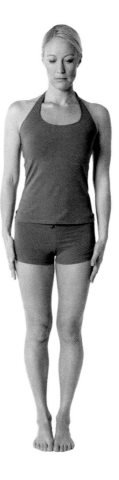

This is the basis for all poses. It is the source of all the branching out of the other asanas. Tadasana brings stability, security, and calm and creates balance, building the stability and strength of the entire body if it is done correctly. Tadasana also helps us to find correct posture. It relieves muscular sciatica and helps flat feet. Don't hold this position for too long if you have a headache, insomnia, or low blood pressure.

Utthita Trikonasana: Extended triangle pose

Utthita = extended; Tri = three; Kona = angle. Trikona = three angles, triangle

1. Stand in Tadasana. Exhale and spread the feet wide, stretch the arms out at the sides, open the chest. The right foot should point straight ahead and the left foot should be at a 90-degree angle. Engage the thighs.

2. Draw the navel in, lift the chest, and drop the shoulders. Stretch out the right arm as far as you can as you inhale.

3. Tip the hip over, toward the thigh, but keep the back straight. Beginners can take a strong hold somewhere below the knee, those with more experience can hold at the ankle or even hold the big toe. Keep the shoulders stacked straight over the left leg, keep the chest lifted, draw the navel toward the spine, keep the right thigh lifted toward the ceiling. Stay in this position and take eight breaths.

Coming out: Exhale, look at the left foot and bend the left knee. On the next inhale let the right arm pull you up, and when you have a straight back look out over the right hand and the middle finger; then reverse the position of the feet to prepare to repeat on the other leg.

Drishti: the palm of the hand
Bandhas: *Mula* and *Uddiyana* bandha

Utthita Trikonasana stretches and strengthens the muscles of hips, legs, lower back, and belly. It develops strength in the upper back, neck, and wrists. The pose relieves stress, aches and pains during menopause, back pains, and improves digestion. Avoid this pose if you have diarrhea or a bad headache. If you have low blood pressure, you should not hold longer than eight breaths if you feel distress; if you suffer from high blood pressure, you can look down instead of up. If you have neck problems, hold the head straight and look down.

Parivritta Trikonasana: Reverse triangle

Paivritta = reversed, turned around/back; Trikonasana = triangle position

Parivritta Trikonasana often follows Utthita Trikonasana. If you come from Tadasana, widen your stance and find the posture for Utthita Trikonasana.

1. Turn the chest over the right leg. Take a steady grip on the hip. Swivel the left foot inward about 45 degrees. Let the hips point straight ahead. Engage the legs, draw in the navel, and lift the chest and shoulders. Breathe in, stretch the back, and look at the right foot.

2. Exhale and lean forward over the right leg. Keep the back straight. Swivel the hip toward the right leg so that the chest points out to the right. Beginners can take hold of the ankle or shin; advanced practitioners can set the hands on the mat outside the foot. Engage the thighs so as not to overstress the knee.

3. Lay the right arm on the lower back and push the chest forward. If you can go further without bending the back, stretch up the right arm and look at the hand. Hold the pose and take 8 deep breaths.

Coming out: Exhale, look down at the right leg and bend the knee. Inhale and follow the right arm up and prepare for the same pose on the opposite leg. Then come back to *Tadasana* and find the breath.

Drishti: the palm of the hand
Bandhas: *Mula* and *Uddiyana* bandha

This is a counterpose to Utthita Trikonasana and is used as a preparation for sitting forward bends and twists. Parivritta Trikonasana shapes and strengthens the waist and legs, strengthens the chest, and reduces lower back problems. It contributes to positive energy and clarity of mind. Don't do this pose if you have intense back or neck problems, or ask for alternatives from your yoga teacher.

Prasarita Padottanasana: Tower pose

Prasarita = outstretched, spread; Pada = foot

From Tadasana: Stand with feet widely spread, hands at your sides, and stretch through the legs. Toes should point straight ahead and heels straight behind. Engage the legs, inhale, and stretch up through the back and the chest. Look up.

1. Exhale and draw the navel in, follow the nose with the gaze forward and down, and fold forward down toward the floor.

2. Inhale and stretch out through the back, follow the tip of the nose with the gaze. Exhale and fall a bit deeper. Stay and breathe. Relax the shoulders, arms, and face.

3. Divide the weight evenly between both legs. If your head does reach the floor, don't bend the neck—keep the spine in a straight line. Press the tongue lightly to the roof of the mouth. Stay here for half a minute and breathe deeply.

Coming out: Reverse the steps that got you into the position, then step feet together to Tadasana.

Drishti: third eye (or close the eyes)
Bandhas: *Mula* and *Uddiyana* bandha

This is an inverted standing pose. Here we are really stretching the legs, especially the back and outside of the thighs. This strengthens the leg muscles, increases movement in the spine, and helps us breathe deeply. In addition, the internal organs of the abdomen are cleansed and revitalized, and stiffness in the neck and shoulders is relieved. This pose is beneficial for digestion; it is helpful for periostitis and helps with inflammation of the Achilles' tendon.

Avoid this pose if you suffer from high blood pressure, ear infection, cataracts, severe asthma, slipped disc, are suffering from a bad cold, or have a very weak back.

Utkatasana: Chair (fierce) pose

Utkana = fire, powerful, fierce

From Tadasana: Stretch the arms up with palms facing each other. Lift the chest, relax the shoulders; look up but don't let the head fall back.

Drishti: thumbs
Bandhas: *Mula* and *Uddiyana* bandha

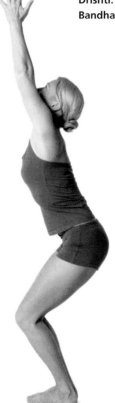

1. Inhale and bend the knees. Exhale, sink the shoulders down the back, lift the chest, and keep the arms and fingers spread.

2. Spread the weight of the body over the entire sole of the foot and press knees together. Step the feet slightly apart and the arms shoulder width apart if that feels better for the neck and the back. Hold the position for 8 breaths.

This positions creates a stretch through the entire body, from the heels to the tips of the fingers. It works the muscles of the arms and legs, and stimulates the heart and the diaphragm. Utkatasana develops movement in the chest, reduces stiffness in the shoulders and chest, and stimulates the inner organs of the stomach, diaphragm, and heart. Don't try to do this exercise if you have a bad headache or intense insomnia. If you have low blood pressure you shouldn't hold this pose for more than four breaths.

Virabhadrasana 1 (A): Warrior 1

Virabhadrasana = the name of a powerful warrior, an incarnation of Shiva

From Tadasana: Take a strong step back with the right foot and set the sole down behind you, maintaining a 45-degree angle. Look out over the left leg, inhale, and lift the hands up over the head so that they meet, at the same time bending the left knee.

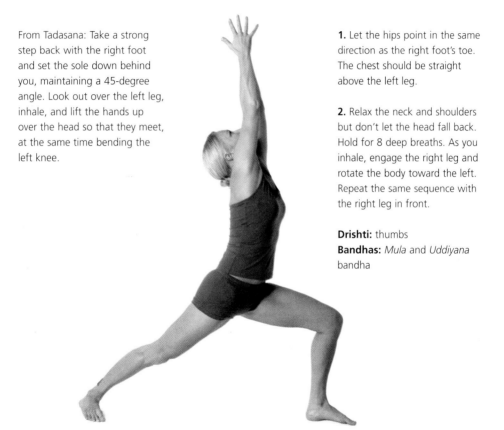

1. Let the hips point in the same direction as the right foot's toe. The chest should be straight above the left leg.

2. Relax the neck and shoulders but don't let the head fall back. Hold for 8 deep breaths. As you inhale, engage the right leg and rotate the body toward the left. Repeat the same sequence with the right leg in front.

Drishti: thumbs
Bandhas: *Mula* and *Uddiyana* bandha

Warrior positions directly increase positive attitudes and give physical control over the body. Keep the back as straight as possible and open the chest. This exercise stretches and strengthens the legs, feet, and ankles, increases flexibility in the hips, chest, and shoulders, and strengthens the lungs. It also stimulates the inner organs of the abdomen and reduces back pain.

Don't do this pose if you suffer from diarrhea or high blood pressure. If you have neck problems you shouldn't look up; look straight ahead, but keep the neck straight.

Virabhadrasana II (B): Warrior 2

Virabhadrasana = the name of a powerful warrior, an incarnation of Shiva

From Tadasana: Take a big step back (a little bit bigger than in Warrior 1) with the right foot, and place the sole of the foot at a 90-degree angle behind you. Look out over the left leg, inhale, and lift the hands straight up over the legs, at the same time bending the left knee.

Drishti: middle finger
Bandhas: *Mula* and *Uddiyana* bandha

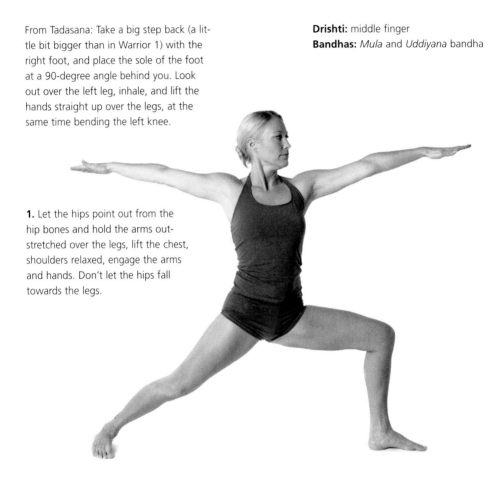

1. Let the hips point out from the hip bones and hold the arms outstretched over the legs, lift the chest, shoulders relaxed, engage the arms and hands. Don't let the hips fall towards the legs.

This exercise strengthens and stretches the legs, feet, and wrists it increases flexibility in the hips, chest, and shoulders and strengthens the lungs. It also reduces back pain and stimulates the inner organs of the abdomen.

Don't do this pose if you suffer from diarrhea or untreated high blood pressure. If you have a neck injury you can look down or straight ahead, but hold the neck straight.

Vrksana: Tree pose

Vrksa = tree

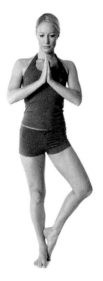

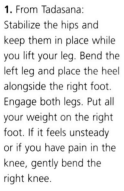

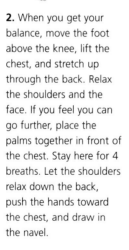

3. Stretch the arms up over the head. Interlace the fingers, except for the index finger and thumb. Hold for 4 breaths. Slowly release the hands down and repeat the same with the right leg. End in Tadasana.

1. From Tadasana: Stabilize the hips and keep them in place while you lift your leg. Bend the left leg and place the heel alongside the right foot. Engage both legs. Put all your weight on the right foot. If it feels unsteady or if you have pain in the knee, gently bend the right knee.

2. When you get your balance, move the foot above the knee, lift the chest, and stretch up through the back. Relax the shoulders and the face. If you feel you can go further, place the palms together in front of the chest. Stay here for 4 breaths. Let the shoulders relax down the back, push the hands toward the chest, and draw in the navel.

Drishti: straight ahead to an unmoving point on the floor, or the tip of the nose if you feel steady
Bandhas: *Mula* and *Uddiyana* bandha

This pose strengthens the legs, back, foot joints, and feet, and improves balance and posture. As with all balancing poses, the drishti is very important.

Don't do this pose if you have a bad headache, intense insomnia, if you suffer from very low blood pressure, or faint easily. If you suffer from high blood pressure you should not lift your arms over your head in this posture.

Natarajasana: Dancing Shiva/Standing bow pose

Nata = dancer; Raja = king

From Tadasana: Set the gaze on an unmoving point on the floor in front of you. Place both hands on the hips and keep this stability with the hips parallel to the floor.

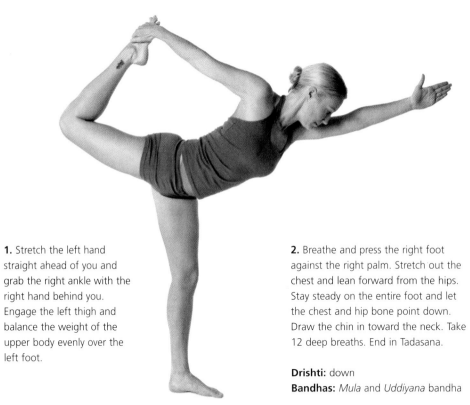

1. Stretch the left hand straight ahead of you and grab the right ankle with the right hand behind you. Engage the left thigh and balance the weight of the upper body evenly over the left foot.

2. Breathe and press the right foot against the right palm. Stretch out the chest and lean forward from the hips. Stay steady on the entire foot and let the chest and hip bone point down. Draw the chin in toward the neck. Take 12 deep breaths. End in Tadasana.

Drishti: down
Bandhas: *Mula* and *Uddiyana* bandha

This position is considered both a standing and a balancing pose and strengthens and develops the muscles of the legs. The flexibility of the shoulder blades is improved and the chest opens. All the vertebrae are favorably stretched. This pose even improves concentration.

Balasana: Child's pose

Bala = Child. Also strong, energetic

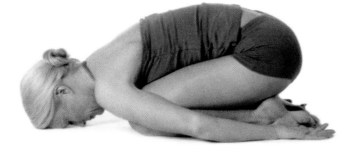

1. Come to all fours with knees hips' distance apart; don't let the toes meet. Sink your seat toward the heels and stretch out the back as much as possible. Lay the forehead to the floor. Stretch the throat and relax the jaw, shoulders, and neck.

2. Let the arms rest alongside the ears or along the body with the palms of the hands facing up. Relax the whole body and feel how the breath fills all the way out into the upper back. Widen the chest as you inhale and let it rest as you exhale.

Drishti: down
Bandhas: *Mula* bandha

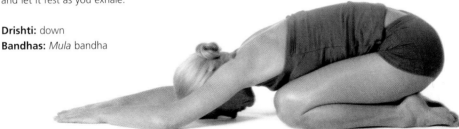

Child's pose is a resting forward bend and is often used between more demanding poses to restore energy and strength. Child's pose is always the counterpose for Ushtrasana (see page 90). This pose increases the circulation of blood to the back and improves flexibility in the hips, thighs, and wrists. It alleviates menstruation discomfort and reduces stress and fatigue. Avoid this pose if you are suffering from diarrhea. If you have problems with the knees you can ask your teacher for variations on this pose.

Paschimottanasana: Full forward bend

Paschimottana = intensive stretch of the front of the body

1. Sit with legs stretched in front of you and a straight back. Flex the feet, engage the front of the thighs, and hold the legs together. Place your hands by either side of the body. Lift the chest and look at the toes. This position is called Dandasana. Stay here for 5 long, deep breaths. Press down through the seat bones and engage the front of the thighs.

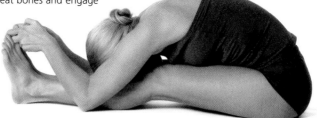

2. Inhale and take a steady hold on the calves. Don't let the chest just fall on to the legs; instead stretch the spine straight up. Stay where you feel resistance. Exhale, engage the thighs, stretch the feet, and draw the back up straighter. Inhale and stretch out the spine, exhale and let gravity do its work.

Drishti: nose tip or eyes closed
Bandhas: *Mula* and *Uddiyana* bandha

3. Take a hold of the feet with the hands or grip the big toe with the thumb and index finger. Relax the shoulders and close the eyes. Stay where it begins to feel difficult and take 12 deep breaths. Come slowly back by first holding the pose and inhaling, then exhale and stretch up through the back, coming to Dandasana.

Paschimottanasana strengthens the legs and abdominal muscles and increases flexibility in the back of the thighs and along the spine—it is an intense back stretch. Primarily the movement stimulates the kidneys, the liver, and the pancreas when you activate the abdomen and breathe with the diaphragm. The pose acts to calm and counteract stress, and relieves menstrual discomfort, headache, and menopause symptoms.

Avoid this pose if you suffer from diarrhea or a slipped disc. If you suffer from severe asthma or back problems you should only practice this position after consulting with an experienced yoga teacher.

Uttanasana: Head against the knees pose

Ute = intensive; Tan = to extend, stretch out

From Tadasana: Stand with feet spread one foot apart. Keep a straight line from the hip bones down to the middle toe. It is important that toes point straight ahead and heels straight back.

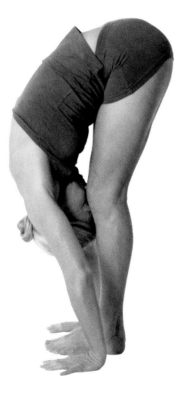

1. Take hold of the lower part of the hips. The weight is spread over the feet.

2. Engage the big toes and the front of the thighs. Lift the chest, roll back the shoulders. Inhale, hold gaze down the tip of the nose, lengthen the back, and gently bend the knees at the same time as you exhale.

3. Fall forward with a straight back. Better to bend the knees and keep the back straight than vice-versa. Let the arms hang down and relax the upper body.

4. Breath calmly and deeply into the throat and the lower part of the chest. Close the eyes, keep the mouth closed, and gently press the tongue to the roof of the mouth. Engage the front of the thighs and relax the back. Hold for 12 deep breaths.

5. If this feels fine, develop Uttanasana by coming to Supta Uttanasana (Resting head to knees pose). Hug the elbows and relax in the neck, shoulders, face; take the final 6 breaths here. Close the eyes or look toward the navel. Control the breath so that it is calm, deep, and long.

Drishti: navel or eyes closed
Bandhas: *Mula* and *Uddiyana* bandha

This pose increases blood circulation to the back side of the body and counteracts depression and stress, improves digestion, relieves symptoms of menopause, reduces fatigue and anxiousness, and helps stop headaches and insomnia.

If you have back problems you can do this position with bent knees or hands on a stool or block for support.

Setu Bandha Sarvangasana: Bridge pose

Setu = bridge; Bandha = lock

1. Lie on your back. Bend the knees and set the soles of the feet against the floor, about hips' distance apart, with the heels close to the back of the thighs. Don't let the knees fall apart. Try to touch the heels with the fingers.

2. Press together the shoulder blades and think about drawing the head softly away from the shoulders. Relax in the neck and look toward the navel. Inhale and hold.

3. Exhale and lift up the buttocks and hips as high as you can. Keep the mouth closed (but relax in the jaw) and lightly press the tongue to the roof of the mouth. Try to get support from the head, neck, shoulders, arms, and feet. Hold for at least 12 deep breaths.

Coming out: Inhale and hold the position, then exhale while you sink down in the hips. Put your weight in the legs coming down. End by lying on your back and hugging the knees to the chest. Feel how the lower back muscles completely relax. Then lie flat.

Drishti: navel
Bandhas: *Mula, Uddiyana,* and *Jalandhara* bandha

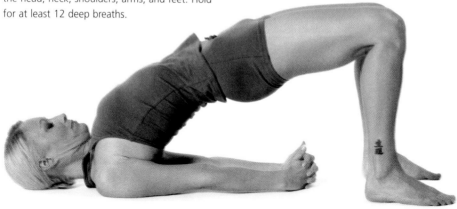

This position is also called Kandharasana (shoulder pose) and is a counterpose to Paschimottanasana and Navasana. Tension is released from the upper back, shoulders, and neck, while flexibility in the chest, neck, and spine increase. This improves digestion, strengthens the female reproductive organs, and is said to reduce asthma.

Avoid this pose if you have neck problems, ulcers, or problems in the stomach area.

Urdhva Dhanurasana: Wheel pose

Urdhva = uplift; Dhanu = bow

1. Lie on your back. Bend the knees and place the feet about a foot apart with the heels facing in toward the buttocks. Make sure the toes point straight ahead and the heels are in line with the body.

2. Place the hands beside the head; the fingers should face in toward the shoulders. Try at the same time to spread the fingers out. Lift up slowly from the floor with power from the legs and arms, using support from the pelvis to carefully bend the spine backward. Keep the head pointing toward the floor. Breathe deep, slow breaths. If you need to, move the hands a little closer together to improve support.

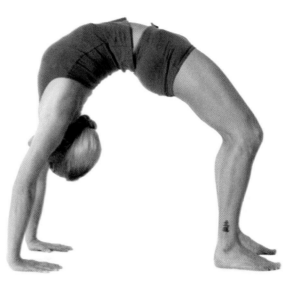

3. Inhale and stretch the arms and legs out as much as you can so that the head and upper body are lifted. Let the head hang between the arms. Lift the heels for a moment and then let them drop. Try to hold this position for 5-12 deep breaths.

To come out: Exhale pushing the weight firmly up through the pelvis, abdominals, legs, and arm muscles. Do this three times if it feels okay. Then rest with the knees to the chest. Balance with a forward bend such as Paschimottanasana (see page 86). Roll to the side and slowly sit up.

Drishti: between the eyebrows
Bandhas: *Mula* bandha

Urdhva Dhanurasana is an advanced position; only do this if you have mastered easier back bends. These asanas are always followed by forward bends in which Halasana (the Plow) and Sarvangasana (Shoulder stand) are good counterposes. This pose strengthens the arms, hand joints, foot joints, legs, seat, abdomen, and spine.

Avoid Urdhva Dhanurasana if you have diarrhea, headache, heart problems, high blood pressure, low blood pressure, very weak hand joints or ankles, or back problems.

Ushtrasana: Camel pose

Ushtra = camel

1. Kneel with the knees hips distance apart. Lean back, reach for the ankles and roll the hips upward at the same time that you lift the chest. Breathe deeply. Beginners can place the hands a bit behind the body and let the fingertips point away from the body.

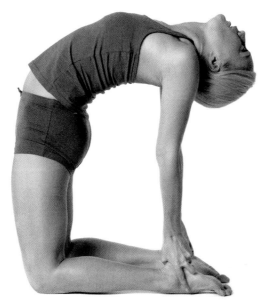

2. Inhale and slowly push away from the soles of the feet. Stay where you meet resistance and keep the legs and pelvis engaged.

3. Look back, lift the chest, and release through the neck. Avoid gripping in the buttocks. Hold the position for 8-12 breaths.

4. Bend gently back while looking up, and try to take a hold of the heels. Hold for 8-12 breaths.

Coming out: Inhale and hold. While you exhale, sink the hips gradually and look slowly down toward the navel, keeping the weight in the legs. When the buttocks reach the heels, straighten the back and breathe in deeply, then come carefully down over the legs while exhaling, coming to Balasana (page 85). Close the eyes and relax in the shoulders. If at any time you feel any sharp pain in the back in this position, stop immediately and come down to rest in Balasana.

Drishti: third eye
Bandhas: *Mula* bandha

Ushtrasana should always be followed by a forward bend. If you get any pain in the knees, place a tightly folded towel under the hollows of the knees during the pose. Ushtrasana relieves tension in the neck and shoulders. It works to strengthen and improve digestion and the reproductive system while stretching the abdominal muscles and relieving knee problems. This pose even improves posture and blood circulation to the face.

Avoid this pose if you suffer from diarrhea, intense back pain, or have an impaired thyroid gland.

Bakasana: Crane pose

Baka = crane

1. Squat with the feet shoulder distance apart. Balance on the balls of the feet directly behind the toes, place the palms of the hands in front of you and slightly to the sides of the feet. Spread the fingers and slightly bend the elbows.

2. Place the knees on top of the backside of the arms. Stretch out the chest and feel that you are supporting yourself through the hands. Breath long, deep breaths.

3. Place more of your weight forward. Keep the buttocks moving up through space while you carefully try to lift one foot and then the other off the floor. Stretch through the feet and try to get the toes to meet. Hold the position for 12 breaths. Don't lose the drishti, even if you lose your balance—keep breathing and relaxing.

Drishti: tip of the nose or the third eye
Bandhas: *Mula* bandha

This position is also called Baka Dhyanasana (Patient crane). Coordination, focus, and technique are required here more than physical strength and flexibility. The pose helps build and strengthen the abdominal organs, lower back, chest, shoulders, and arms, and adds flexibility to the shoulder blades, foot joints, and toes. Avoid this pose if you suffer from high blood pressure, heart problems, or you have eye problems.

Pada Angushthasana: Toe balance

Pada = foot; Angushtha = thumb/toe

1. Squat, with hands at your sides, focus the gaze on a point in front of you. Stretch up through the back and lift the chest. Keep the breath even, deep, and slow.

2. Lift the heels and balance on the toes. Push the thighs forward so that they maintain a horizontal line. Stay sitting on the toes and keep the back straight. Let the palms come together at the chest and relax the shoulders. Hold the position for 12 breaths.

3. Then inhale and hold, exhale and carefully stand up, bend forward to come slowly into Uttanasana (see page 87). Hold the position for 4 deep breaths.

Drishti: tip of the nose or straight ahead
Bandhas: *Mula* or *Uddiyana* bandha

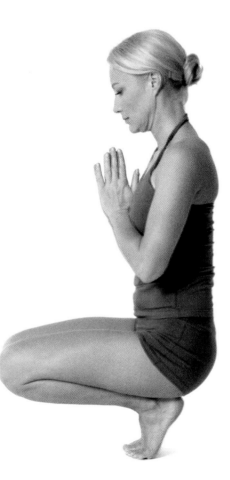

This asana helps to develop concentration and focus as well as to open the mind. It strengthens the feet and increases blood circulation to the thighs and legs. It increases balance and builds flexibility in the legs, joints of the feet, and the toes. It improves balance and decreases flat feet.

If you have severe knee problems you should ask your yoga teacher to modify the pose for you.

Parivritta Utkatasana: Revolved fierce pose

Parivritta = revolved; Taka = fire, glowing, fierce

1. Squat with hands at your sides and fasten your gaze at a point in front of you. Stretch through the back and lift the chest. Breathe evenly, deeply, and slowly.

2. Place your hands together at your chest. Relax in your shoulders and keep your shoulder blades and chest engaged.

3. Inhale and hold the position, exhale and twist the top of the body to the left, setting the right elbow to the outside of the left thigh. Drop the shoulders and carefully stretch the neck. Follow the movement with your gaze.

4. Stretch the head out from the shoulders and press the palms together. Press down through the big toes. Don't hang over the legs with the upper body. Stretch out through the back. Hold the position for 8-12 breaths.

To come out: Inhale and hold the position, exhale and slowly drop the gaze and look to the right. Let the upper body follow. Then repeat the movement on the other side. Come slowly to Uttanasana (see page 87). Hold the position for 8 deep breaths.

Drishti: up toward the sky
Bandhas: *Uddiyana* bandha

Parivritta Utkatasana is both a twist and a balancing pose. Here the legs, back, abdomen, neck, and chest are strengthened. The pose increases blood circulation through the entire body it releases stress from the vertebrae, discs, and nerves of the spine, and counteracts constipation and improves digestion. It is beneficial for mental balance.

Avoid this pose if you suffer from severe menstrual pains or if you are suffering from slipped discs.

Ardha Matsyendrasana: Sitting spinal twist

Ardha = half; Matsyendra = Fisherman's king (matsya = fish)

1. Sit in Dandasana, see page 86.

2. Lift the right foot over the top of the left leg, toward the buttocks. Divide your weight evenly over the seat bones. Hug your right knee with the left arm and set the right hand behind the sacrum, fingers pointing away from the body.

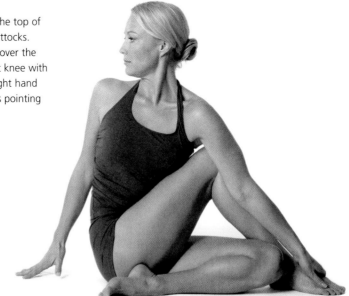

3. Inhale and straighten up through the back, pushing the right knee toward the left armpit with the left arm. Angle the palm of the hand and spread the fingers. Exhale and open the trunk to the right so that you are looking over the right shoulder. Hold the position for 12 deep breaths. Reverse position and twist to the left.

Drishti: Parsva, to the horizon
Bandhas: *Mula* and *Uddiyana* bandha

This is a very effective asana but requires the right technique for maximum effect. It increases blood circulation, flexibility, and strength in the spinal muscles and neck muscles, supports digestion, and lowers body stress. It relieves menstruation pains, fatigue, and sciatica. Avoid this position if you have ulcers. If you have extreme back problems you should only do this under the supervision of an experienced yoga teacher.

Ardha Rajakapotasana: Half pigeon pose

Ardha = half; Raja = king; Kapota = dove, pigeon

1. From Parvatasana (see page 60) inhale and press the right knee forward toward the right hand. Place the right lower leg in as close to a right angle as possible under you, so that the right sole of the foot lands to the outside of the left arm.

2. Place the hands on either side of the right leg, straighten the left leg out behind you. Divide the weight of the body evenly. Inhale, look up, and stretch through the back, exhale and sink down, bringing the elbows to the floor.

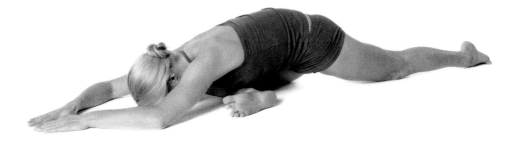

3. Hold the back straight and relax in the shoulders. Focus the gaze right in front of you. Inhale and move forward slowly with the hands. Stay where you meet resistance, close your eyes, relax and take 10-20 long and deep breaths.

Then return to Parvatasana and stretch out. Change legs, or go to Eda Pada Rajakapotasana (see next page).

Drishti: tip of the nose or close the eyes
Bandhas: *Mula* and *Uddiyana* bandha

Pigeon contains five different variations, of which the most common are: half pigeon, one-legged pigeon, and full pigeon. Pigeon strengthens the hips and increases flexibility and balance in the pelvis, hips, buttocks, and lower back. It is also an effective stretch of the backside, outside of the thighs, and lower back. It strengthens both the muscle tissue and the muscle itself. Pigeon is considered a sitting position, as well as a resting pose and even a forward bend. Half pigeon stretches the buttocks muscles, outside of the thighs, groin, upper back, and shoulders.

Eka Pada Rajakapotasana: One-legged pigeon

Eka = one; Pada = foot, leg; Raja = king; Kapota = pigeon

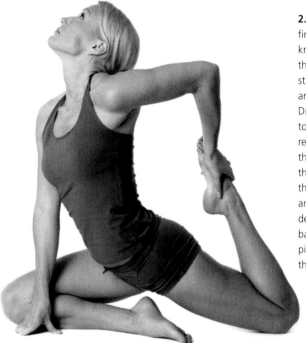

2. Set down the right knuckles or fingertips on the inside of the right knee and push off the hand. Lift the gaze and hold the neck straight. Gently bend the left leg and take a hold of the left ankle. Draw the foot in toward the buttock at the same time that you use resistance, pressing the foot into the hand. Bend the elbow and roll the shoulders back. Avoid swaying the back, work to keep the arms and legs engaged. Breathe 8-12 deep breaths then come gently back into Parvatasana. Repeat Half pigeon and One-legged pigeon on the other side.

1. Instead of changing the leg in Ardha Rajakapotasana you can do Eka Pada Rajakapotasana on the same side to deepen the pose. Raise yourself up on straight arms. Draw in the right foot so that the heel is under the left groin. Raise the right hip off the ground.

Drishti: third eye or looking up to the sky
Bandhas: *Mula* or *Uddiyana* bandha

One-legged pigeon stretches the inside and outside of the thighs, groin, abdomen, chest, shoulders, and neck. The pose stimulates the internal abdominal organs and increases circulation to the pelvis and hips.

Avoid this pose if you have severe knee or foot problems.

Navasana: Boat pose

Nava = boat

1. From a seated position: Inhale, bend the knees and draw them up toward the chest. Hug the knees with the hands and straighten the back. Lean back so that you are balancing on your seat bones. Stretch up through the back. Keep the legs together and hold under the knees with the hands. Breathe and lift up one leg at a time.

2. Engage the fronts of the thighs. Straighten the arms so that they are parallel over the legs. Engage the hands and keep the fingers together except for the thumb, which should point up. Divide your weight between the seat bones and the tail bone. Hold this position for 5 breaths. Keep the back straight and don't sacrifice your posture in order to keep the legs straight.

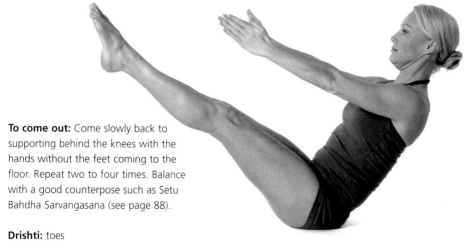

To come out: Come slowly back to supporting behind the knees with the hands without the feet coming to the floor. Repeat two to four times. Balance with a good counterpose such as Setu Bahdha Sarvangasana (see page 88).

Drishti: toes
Bandhas: *Mula* and *Uddiyana* bandha

This is extremely good for building strength in the back, legs, and abdominals. Navasana strengthens the belly, trunk, and upper back and stimulates the kidneys, pancreas, pituitary gland, and the intestines. It relieves stress and improves digestion. Avoid this pose if you suffer from diarrhea, severe headaches, heart problems, or if you have severe insomnia. You should also avoid this during the first 2–3 days of menstruation. If you have a neck injury, rest your head against a wall when you lift up your legs.

Virasana: Hero pose

Vira = person, hero, leader

1. Sit back on the knees. Hold the knees together and move the feet out to the sides of the hips. Lift the seat from the feet and sink back with the buttocks between the feet. Place the hands on the knees and look at the navel. Stay here as long as you can, at least 12 breaths (you might feel a big pull through the legs but try to breathe through it). Then stretch out in Parvatasana (see page 60).

Drishti: tip of the nose
Bandhas: *Mula* and *Uddiyana* bandha

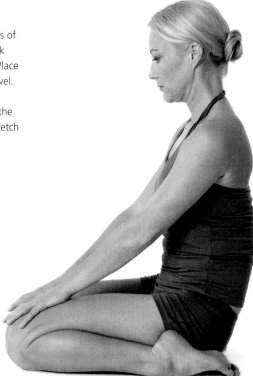

This pose is good to do after eating as it balances digestion. Supta Virasana (resting hero, see photo at right) stretches the stomach muscles, hips, knees, foot joints, groin, and front of the thighs. These two asanas are very effective to resolve knee problems. If you experience pain during the pose, fold a towel tightly and lay it under the hollow of the knees. This pose strengthens the arches and relieves menopause symptoms. Avoid this position if you suffer from heart problems, severe headaches, or have knee or ankle joint injuries.

Supta Virasana: Resting hero pose

Vira = person, hero, leader

1. Place the hands behind the back and prepare for Supta Virasana (resting hero). Lean back a little, but not enough to be swaybacked. If it feels okay, go down on the elbows, take a hold of the feet with the hands, relax the neck, lift the chest, and lay the crown of the head on the floor.

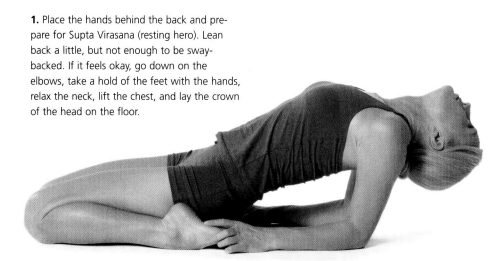

2. Lay the top of the back down with the hands overhead and take hold of the elbows. Relax and breathe deeply and calmly. Avoid separating the knees too much—no more than hips' distance apart, with the goal being to keep them touching.

Drishti: down the tip of the nose
Bandhas: *Mula* and *Uddiyana* bandha

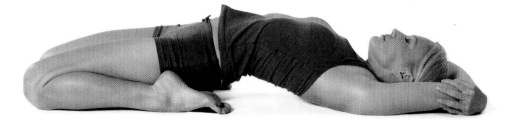

Baddha Konasana: Butterfly pose

Baddha = bound; Kona = angle

1. From a sitting position: Inhale, press feet against each other, and draw the heels in toward the pelvis. Stay on your seat bones. Stretch up through the spine. Take a hold of the feet, interlacing the fingers, and slowly press the knees toward the floor. Inhale and push the chest forward and relax in the hips and shoulders. Exhale.

2. If you are an experienced yoga practitioner you can then bend over the legs without bending in the back or bringing the legs toward the ears, place the forehead to the floor, and take 8 deep breaths. Try to maintain a straight spine and work to keep good posture while the knees are pressing down.

Drishti: tip of the nose
Bandhas: *Mula* and *Uddiyana* bandha

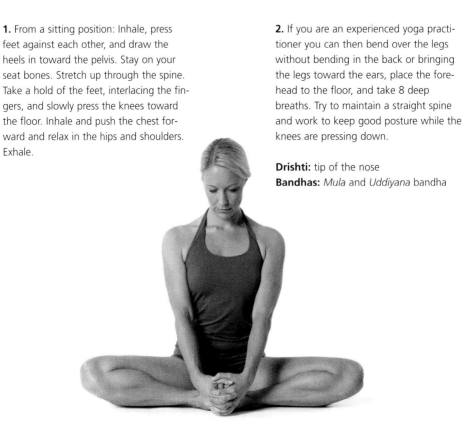

The increased blood flow from Baddha Konasana cleanses the pelvic region, the lower portion of the abdomen, and back. It relieves varicose veins, constipation, and digestive problems. It increases movement in the hip joints, groin, knees, thighs, and along the spine. Baddha Konasana also stretches the groin, the front of the thighs, and the muscles of the hips. The pose can also counteract mild depression, anxiety, and fatigue and reduce menstruation discomfort, menopause symptoms, and sciatica. If you have injuries in the groin or the knees, you should only do this pose using a support for the back side of the thighs.

Upavishta Konasana: Seated angle pose

Upavishta = upright; Kona = angle

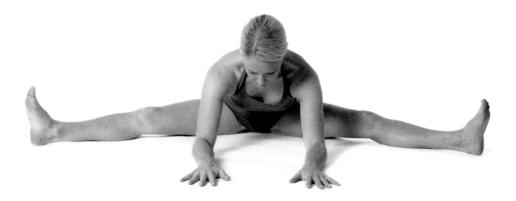

1. Sit with a straight back and legs straight ahead. Place the hands under the buttocks muscles and move the flesh back a bit. Straighten the back and let the legs come apart to make a "V." Stretch out the feet and engage the front of the thighs, toes pointing upward. Push the chest forward. Inhale and push forward with the seat bones. Focus on the breath and posture and let the body do its work.

2. Keep the trunk stretched and stable as you inhale, fall forward with a straight back as you exhale. Close your eyes and continue for 25 breaths. If you want more of a challenge, try to grip the feet.

To come out: Inhale and hold the pose; while exhaling, bring the back slowly upright to sitting and draw the legs together.

Drishti: tip of the nose
Bandhas: *Mula* bandha

In this pose both the legs and the abdominal muscles are strengthened, and flexibility in the back side of the thighs and along the spine is increased. The back, the thighs, and the buttocks are intensively stretched. The forward movement stimulates the kidneys, liver, and the pancreas, as you are activating a belly support as well as breathing with the diaphragm. In addition, with practice this pose releases stress in the shoulders and chest. Remember that if you suffer from severe lower back problems you should consult an experienced yoga teacher before you do the pose.

Padmasana: Lotus pose

Padma = lotus

1. Ardha padmasana (half-lotus): Sit cross-legged, lift and straighten the spine, sink the shoulders down the back, and engage the upper back. Place the right sole of the foot under the inside of the left thigh. Lay the left foot at the bend of the right knee.

2. Padmasana: Lift the right foot in and up toward the left groin so that the foot rests on the left thigh. Then take a hold of the left foot and place it toward the right groin. Try to press the knees a little toward one another. Place the hands in a chosen *mudra* (see pages 31-33).

The road to lotus pose can seem long, but start with a good control of tailor pose (Sukhasana) — rather than crossing your legs, simply allow the soles of your feet to meet in front of you — and then move on to Ardha padmasana.

Keep the spine straight and sit comfortably, even on a pillow, folded blanket, or yoga mat to raise the buttocks slightly.

Drishti: tip of the nose
Bandhas: Mula, Uddiyana or Jalandhara bandha

This pose improves your balance, it is calming, and it stretches out the joints of the feet and the knees while increasing the flexibility of the pelvis, spine, and abdomen. It relieves menstrual pain and sciatica. Padmasana is seen as a medium-difficult to difficult pose. Don't try it without the instruction of an experienced yoga teacher. Do Ardha padmasana (half-lotus) instead, until you feel you can maintain the pose for a while, before moving on.

Halasana: Plow pose

Hala = plow

1. Lie on your back with the knees in to the chest, arms alongside the body. Inhale and lift up the feet a bit. Exhale and press down in the palms of the hands and stretch through the back. Place the hands on the lower back. Stretch the throat. Close the mouth and press the tongue to the roof of the mouth. Bend the hips at the groin and slowly sink the legs down over the body. Try to place the toes behind the head, but keep the back straight.

2. Stretch through the legs and interlace the fingers behind the back and keep them pressed down. Go up onto the tops of the shoulder blades and try to keep the weight on the top half of the shoulder blades.

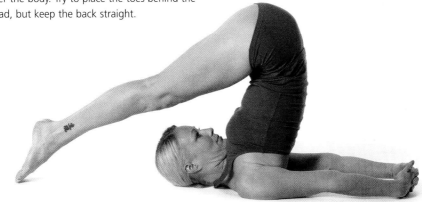

To come out: Place the hands back onto the lower back. Bend the knees and fold them toward the chest. Open the arms and place them alongside the body. Keep the abdominals tight and roll down onto the spine. Carefully swing the body from side to side until you feel the back muscles relaxing.

Drishti: tip of the nose
Bandhas: *Mula* and *Jalandhara* bandha

This is a whole body stretch that increases movement in the spinal column and strengthens the legs and abdominal muscles. It reduces back pain and can help you to sleep better. It strengthens the abdominal muscles, increases blood circulation, and activates digestion.

Avoid this pose if you suffer from back injuries, slipped disc, high blood pressure, sciatica, or have other serious back problems or joint pain in the neck.

Salamba Sirsasana: Head stand

Salamba = with support (sa = with, alamba = support); Sirsa = head

Please note: if you are unsure of this pose don't do it alone—make sure someone experienced is spotting you. Keep the breath deep and controlled, close the mouth without biting together with the teeth, press the tongue lightly into the roof of the mouth.

1. Fold a blanket and place it in front of you. Sit on the knees with the hands on the legs, buttocks resting on the heels. Bend forward and place the underside of the arms onto the blanket and interlace the fingers in front of you. Place the head on the blanket right behind the interlaced fingers—make sure the head is well supported.

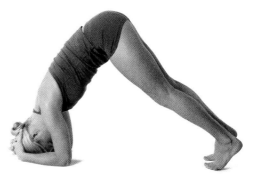

2. Lift up the knees and stretch out the legs. Lift yourself with your arms and shoulder blades and keep the neck supported.

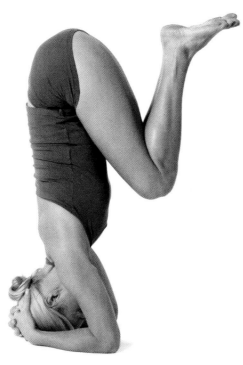

3. Walk your feet forward—get as close to the body as possible. Gently bend the legs and draw the thighs up and in toward the chest and belly. Move the body weight from the toes to the head and arms, try to find balance. Raise the legs approximately 8 inches from the floor, trying to keep your balance. Keep the legs together and the movements slow, and maintain straight posture from the head to the pelvis.

4. Slowly bend the knees and try to let the calves press more closely toward the back of the thighs. Find strength through the lower back and abdominal muscles to find the right positioning.

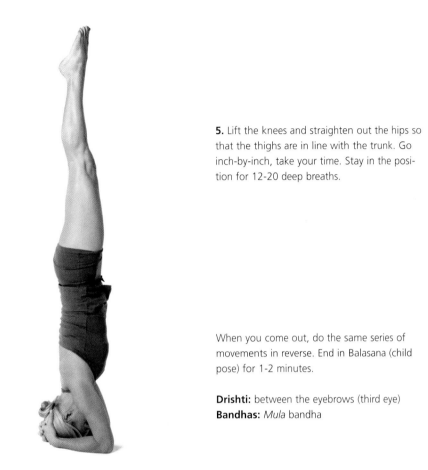

5. Lift the knees and straighten out the hips so that the thighs are in line with the trunk. Go inch-by-inch, take your time. Stay in the position for 12-20 deep breaths.

When you come out, do the same series of movements in reverse. End in Balasana (child pose) for 1-2 minutes.

Drishti: between the eyebrows (third eye)
Bandhas: *Mula* bandha

This asana calms the brain and strengthens the entire body. Sirsasana is called the king of the asanas because it helps to open Sahasrara chakra, the crown chakra, and it stabilizes the pituitary gland. Beginners should always undertake the head stand at the end of the asana training, while more experience practitioners can do it either in the beginning or the middle of a practice. Beginners can work up to four breaths and gradually work up to two more breaths each week if everything feels good.

This pose reduces anxiety, asthma, congestion, insomnia, and symptoms of menopause. It increases blood circulation in the entire body, strengthens the spinal column, and helps the body to fully relax.

Avoid this pose if you have high blood pressure, heart disease, chronic constipation, kidney problems, severe nearsightedness, weak blood vessels in the eyes, or an ear infection.

Salamba Sarvangasana: Shoulder stand

Salamba = with support; Sarva = all; Anga = limbs, extremities

1. Lie on your back and breathe calmly. Lift up the legs, keep them pressed together, try to bring the back up into the air and set the hands at the lower back.

2. Slowly straighten the legs and point the toes, then carefully straighten the body. Keep the mouth closed, without biting the teeth together, and press the tongue to the roof of the mouth. Relax the shoulders, neck, and throat. Take 12 deep breaths.

To come out: Slowly bend the legs and roll slowly down onto the back. Keep the abdominals tight. If you feel discomfort in the back let the hands help. Sink down, lie on the back, and bring the knees to the chest. Hug the knees with the hands. Have a blanket to support the neck if that feels better. Rest in Shavasana (see page 108) until the breath is calm again.

Drishti: toes, tip of the nose, or close the eyes
Bandhas: *Mula* and *Jalandhara* bandha

This position is often called queen of the yoga asanas. There are many positive effects of this pose, among them balancing the thyroid and reducing colds and sinus infections. It has a positive effect on blood circulation, breathing, and digestion. It counteracts stress and headaches. It strengthens the legs and the abdomen and gives increased flexibility to the neck and shoulders. Beginners should only hold this position for a few seconds.

This pose should be avoided by those who have high blood pressure, as well as those who have weak blood vessels in the eyes, and during the first 2–3 days of menstruation.

Matsyasana: Fish pose

Matsya = fish

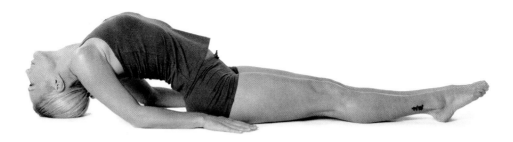

1. Lie outstretched on your back. Press the legs together and point the toes. Let first the right and then the left arm glide under the back. Press the shoulder blades together and sink the buttocks down to rest on the hands. Bend the elbows so that you are balancing on the elbows and the hands. Slowly set the crown of the head onto the floor.

2. Lift the chest. Press through the elbows and relax the shoulders. Press up through the chest as much as possible and breathe deep, calm breaths. Hold for 12 deep breaths. Then carefully come down onto the back and neck.

Drishti: third eye
Bandhas: *Mula* and *Uddiyana* bandha

Here we are working and defining the abdominal, leg, and back muscles. Tension in the neck and the shoulders is released. Blood circulation in the face increases and lung capacity is increased by opening up the chest. This is a counterpose to Salamba Sarvangasana and Halasana and is important to achieve maximum balance in the body. Matsyasana helps most stomach ailments and can relieve constipation (drink three glasses of water and then practice this pose). In addition, it is stimulating for the immune system and relieves back pain.

Avoid this exercise if you suffer from heart disease, ulcers, or disc or other back injuries.

Shavasana: Corpse pose

Shava = like

1. Lie outstretched with arms beside the body, palms facing up. Let the tailbone sink down and lift the chin slightly. Press the heels together and let the feet fall open. Take a deep breath and close the eyes. Breathe long, deep breaths.

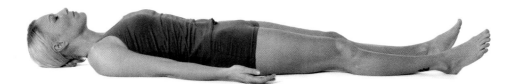

2. Feel how the body sinks down into the floor. Reward yourself with some minutes of complete rest. Continue to breathe and let the muscles keep relaxing. Breathe deeply; the mind is also resting.

3. Tense through the feet when you inhale and then completely relax them when you exhale. Do the same with the hands and feel how you relax more completely in the rest of the body. Now try to relax the face, and continue to breathe. Stay in this resting position for some minutes, optimally 7-15 minutes.

Another name for this asana is Mrtasana (mrta = death). This is a completely relaxing pose, which actually makes it one of the hardest positions in yoga. This pose gives relaxation to the entire body, counteracts stress, and relieves headache and insomnia. It also lowers blood pressure and improves body awareness.

If you suffer from back injuries or feel strong discomfort in this position, you can try bending the knees, keeping the feet on the floor hip-width apart. Use pillows to give the legs support.

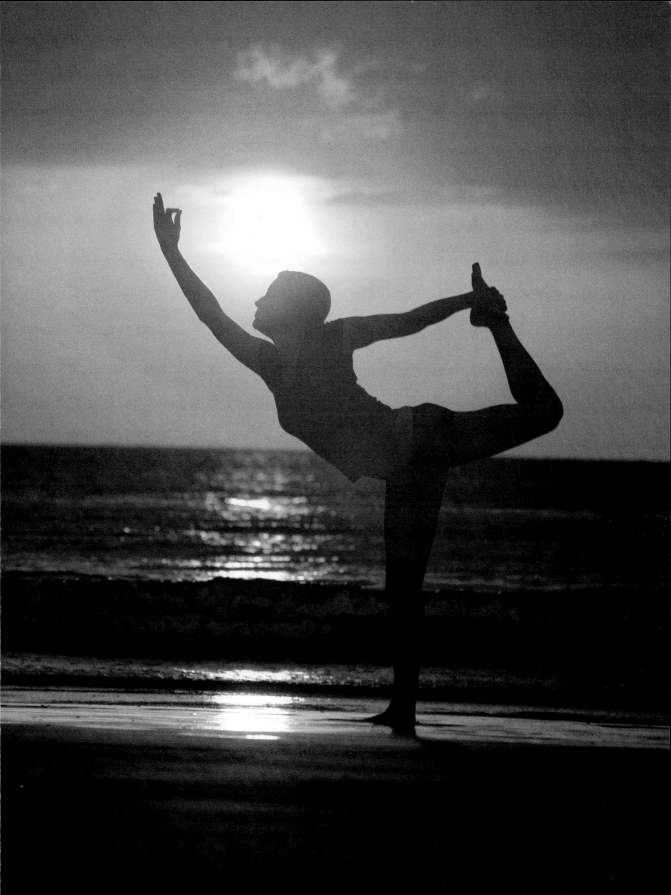

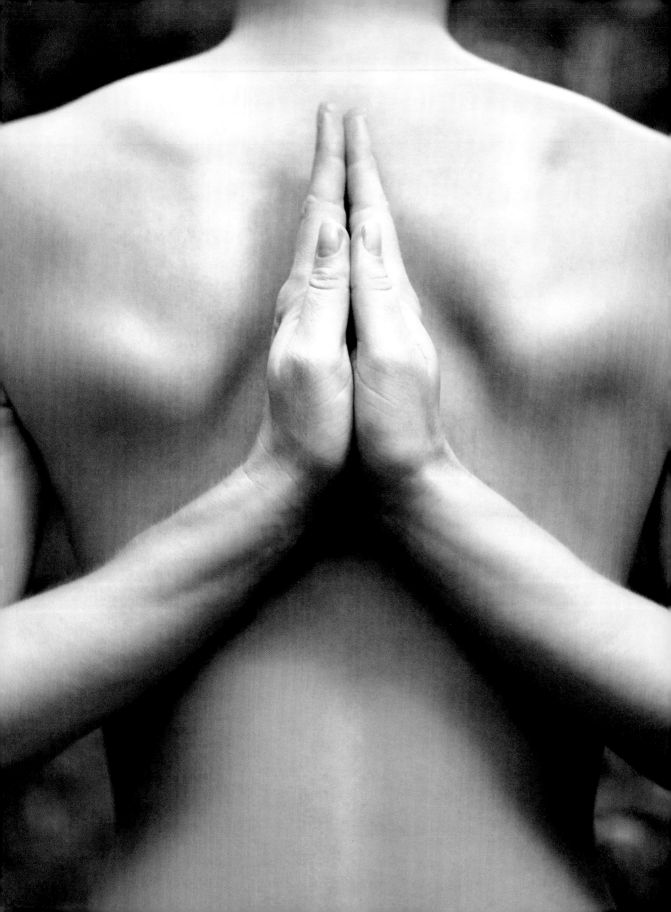

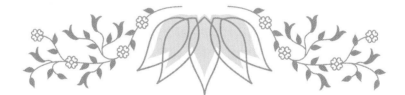

training program

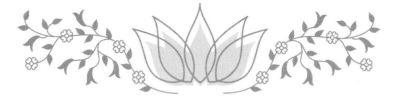

The goal in practicing asanas is to strive for a feeling of calm while challenging yourself. One way to strengthen your energy rather than undermining it is to keep a positive connection with your breath. If you experience active, conscious, and flowing breath and feel active and strong and relaxed—well, then you are on the right track and at the right level of exertion. Remember to listen to your body and breathe. It should never include stabbing pain, although a bit of tingling, pulsing, or pulling is okay and expected.

If you feel too much resistance and the poses feel mentally and spiritually taxing, you should stay at the level that you have reached and focus a bit more on the breath. Concentrate of whether you are relaxing after a breath or two. If the feeling of resistance gets worse in spite of how much effort you expend and it isn't working, come out of the pose and rest in balasana, Child pose. When this happens during an asana, be aware that this is a pose that you will need to come back to again and again. It is pretty important to let this concept really sink in, because as human beings we have a tendency to rush forward as fast as possible just because we think we should or we *can*. What we feel and sense, and what we discover in the body, shows us where we are in life.

On the following pages there are two suggested yoga practice programs. Both examples are fine for beginners, but will work for everyone regardless of yoga experience. The combinations of asanas in these two programs are aimed toward strengthening posture and developing the breath, focus, and concentration. From a wider perspective they will, after regular practice, even contribute to better relaxation and to increased strength and flexibility.

This program is an example of what, within classic Hatha Yoga, is called *sukshma vyayama*, or subtle training. What this means is that negative stress is released from the spinal column and the back, and the hips get stronger, establishing a better base for the free flow of energy to mind and body. Blocked energy in the body is caused all too commonly by bad posture, poorly functioning body processes, emotional issues, or an unbalanced lifestyle. This appears as stiffness, tight muscles, poor blood circulation, and other problems with the functioning of the body's organs. If these blockages become chronic, they often lead to parts of the body becoming weakened, or increased weakness or causing illnesses. The reason to do these asanas is that afterward you feel more balanced in body and soul and your energy is restored—your prana is improved. You shouldn't feel wiped out. This means you've forced the breath, pushed your way through the program, or stressed yourself out, working too hard or too long in some of the positions.

Both programs start with a meditation on the breath, pranayama (see pages 39-47). This should take around 5-10 minutes. After, I have suggested sun or moon salutations (depending on the time of day they are done) as a warm-up and breath expansion. Then some standing, sitting, and cool-down poses follow. How many breaths you should take in each respective asana varies. In general the following recommendations from classic Hatha Yoga apply:

8 breaths for physical stability and development (good for beginners)

12 breaths for physical/mental stamina and strength training (good for when you have mastered the poses and have control of both the breath and the bandhas).

12–21 breaths for mental and spiritual development, strength, and stamina (this will be appropriate when you look at asanas and breath work as a natural part of your day, after some time practicing. In general this takes a couple of years of regular practice).

The program should take around 30 minutes if you hold each position for 8 breaths, but if you want to you can spend more time either at the beginning or at the end in breathwork, or increase the breath time in some poses or lengthen the relaxation if you feel the need. If a pose gives you strong discomfort, simplify or skip that particular one for now. Then consult with your yoga teacher or body worker to find out why you experience the pose in that way.

Hope you have a harmonious time on the mat!

Surya namaskara: Sun salutation

*These twelve positions should be practiced once on each leg,
which constitutes a complete sun salutation.*

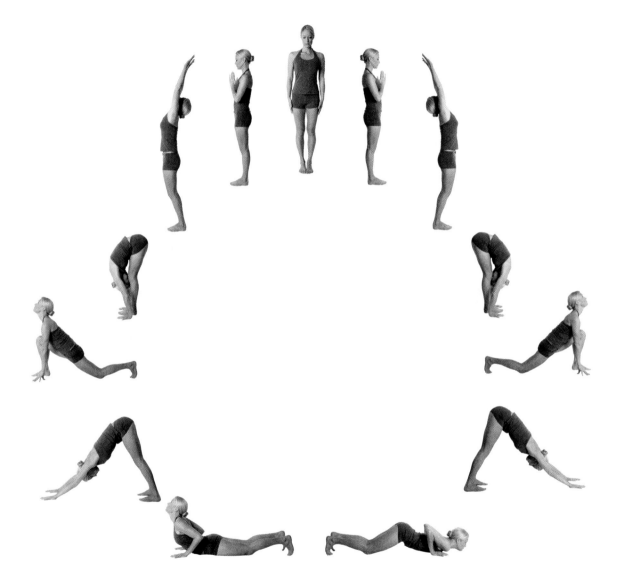

Chandra namaskara: Moon salutation

As with the sun salutation, a complete moon salutation entails a round of the positions on each leg.

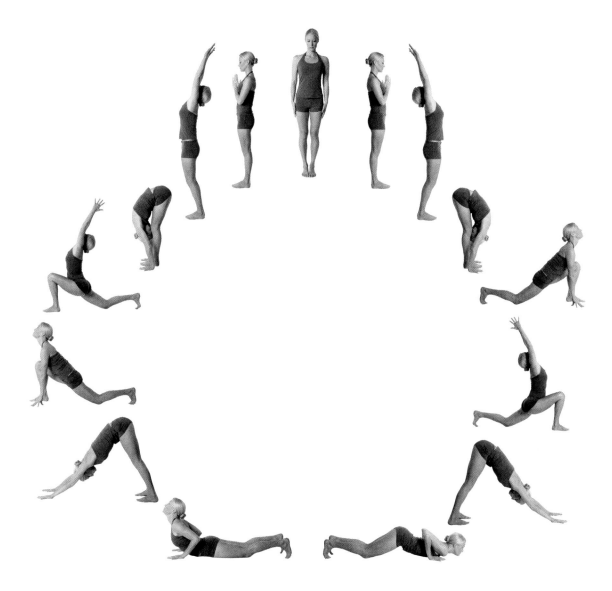

Basic training

*This works morning, noon, or night. If you do these in the evening,
do moon salutations instead of sun salutations.*

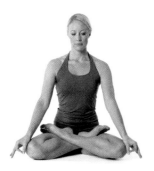
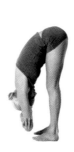
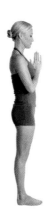
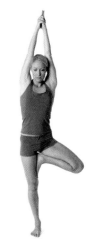

PRANAYAMA

1. *Padmasana*
(introduction and end)

CALMING POSE

2. *Uttanasana*

WARMING POSE

3. *Pranamasana*

STANDING POSE

4. *Vrksana*

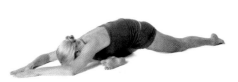
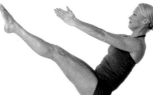
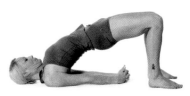

FORWARD BEND

8. *Ardha Rajakapotasana*

SITTING POSE

9. *Navasana*

BACK BEND

10. *Setu Bandha Sarvangasana*

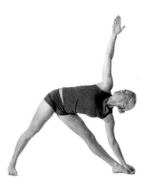

STANDING POSE

5. Utthita Trikonasana

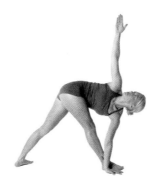

STANDING POSE

6. Parivirtta Trikonasana

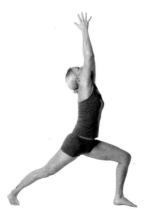

STANDING POSE

7. Virabhadrasana A

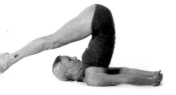

INVERSION

11. Halasana

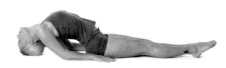

RESTING POSE

12. Matsyasana

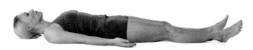

RESTING POSE

13. Shavasana

Gentle hatha

This program is best suited for morning or evening practice.
The recommended number of breaths for asanas 4-14 is between 8-12.

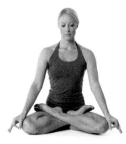

PRANAYAMA
1. *Padmasana (introduction and end)*

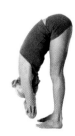

CALMING POSE
2. *Supta uttanasana*

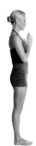

WARMING POSE
3. *Surya/Chandra Namaskara*

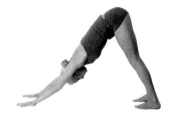

STANDING POSE
7. *Parvatasana*

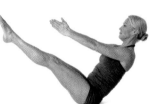

SITTING POSE
8. *Navasana*

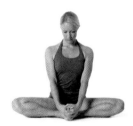

SITTING POSE
9. *Baddha Konasana*

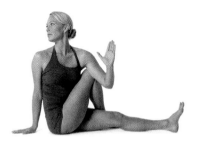

SITTING POSE
12. *Ardha Matsyendrasana*

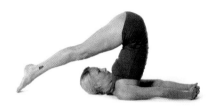

INVERSION
13. *Halasana*

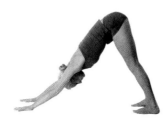

STANDING POSE

4. Parvatasana

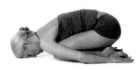

FORWARD BEND

5. Balasana

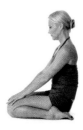

SITTING POSE

6. Virasana

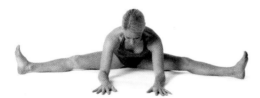

SITTING POSE

10. Upavishta Konasana

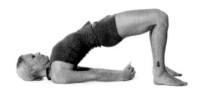

BACK BEND

11. Setu Bandha Sarvangasana

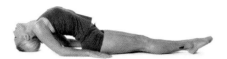

RESTING POSE

14. Matsyasana

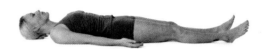

RELAXATION

15. Savasana

Afterword

Asanas and pranayama, along with bandhas, drishti, and mudra, create a training that sharpens the senses. Often Hatha Yoga is defined as "meditation in motion" and this means that before the mind can be really strong and balanced, we have to help it find a safe home to live in—our body. When we have form, body, and mind as one we can see our contents, our soul. It is then that our true spirit is ready to make itself known to us; kundalini (life force). The three development phases—body, mind, and spiritual development—represent the path to yoga. By incorporating awareness into everything we do, our consciousness transforms to wisdom and we develop *Bhumi*, understanding of who we are, why we are, and what we are.

Yoga doesn't make demands based on achievement, perfection, or results. Instead you can be who you are, reveal what you want of yourself, have a great time, and work at your own pace. Yoga gives us power to keep going with less unnecessary strain (also without getting lazy or slow) and even perhaps achieve better results, free from blockages, obstacles, uncertainty, and stress. As a bonus we get the physical benefits, such as muscle development, increased flexibility, better balance, blood circulation, and oxygenation, as well as a balanced metabolism. Our individual requirements play into how each one of us develops. A good piece of advice is to try to avoid results, just do the practice; just do it and keep doing it and see what happens. You'll be undoubtedly and positively surprised.

For me yoga is a great path to self-improvement. These methods have taught me and still teach me to stay present to life and in everything I take on. Even if I practice and teach in more than one yoga form (even Ashtanga Vinyasa Yoga and Power Yoga) it is still classic Hatha Yoga that I consider to be my main branch of practice, as it was here I started my yoga journey. One feeling that grows stronger with each passing day is that I will never give up classic Hatha Yoga, as I can grow old together with it—it gives me more depth and breadth in its dimensions than its branches do.

To write a book about Hatha Yoga is no easy task, as the yogic path to balance has so very many dimensions, structures, and profundities. One can easily become over-ambitious. So we have strived to find a simple structure for the contents, so that they may work as both inspiration and education for you as the reader. Perhaps you actually are enticed into wanting to learn more about Hatha Yoga and yoga in general. Regardless what significance you ascribe to what you have read, I want to wish you the best of luck on your path through life.

And now I want to thank the following people:

My husband, daughter, and family for their love, encouragement, and support. A big thanks as well to Alexandra and Andreas for the time you took to so delicately nuance my words and vision with the book.

I would also like to send a big thanks to Sara Granström, Catarina Falklind-Breschi, Carola Solem, Carina Schutt, Sarah Jonsson, Jan Altersten, Eva Bratt, and all of my teachers and students, as well as all of those who work in the studios where I have taught and now teach.

Om Sri Guru Bhyoh Namaha,

Ulrica

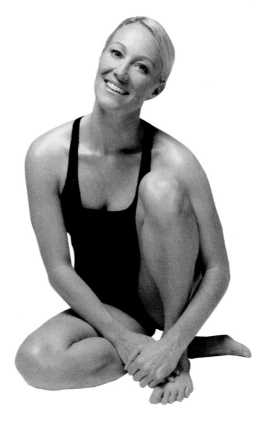

references

Anodea, Judith. *Eastern Body, Western Mind*. Celestial Arts. Berkeley (California, USA), 1996

Coulter, David H. *Anatomy of Hatha Yoga: A Manual for Students, Teachers and Practitioners* Bodyandbreathbooks, 2003

Desikachar, T.K.V. & Cravens R.H. *Health Healing and Beyond: Yoga & The Living Tradition of Krishnamacharya*. Aperture Foundation, 1998

Desikachar, T.K.V. *The Heart of Yoga: Developing a Personal Practice*. Inner Traditions International. Rochester, Vermont, 1995

Feuerstein, Georg & Miller, Jeanine. *The Essence of Yoga*. Inner Traditions. USA, 1998

Iyengar, B.D.S. *Light on Yoga*. Thorsons Aquarian Press, 1991. First published by George Allen & Unwin. Ltd., 1966, 1968, and 1976

Johari, Harish. *Chakras, Energy Centers of Transformation*. Destiny's Books. USA, 1987

Jois, Sri K. Pattabhi. *Yoga Mala*. Patanjali Yoga Shala. New York, 1999

Lalvani, Vimla. *Classic Yoga*. Hamlyn Publishing, London, 1996

Prana Pranayama Prana Vidya. Yoga Publications Trust (Bihar School of Yoga), 2002

Saraswati, Satyananda Swami. *Asana Pranayama Mudra Bandha*, Yoga Publications Trust (Bihar School of Yoga), 1969

Satchidananda, Sri Swami. *The Living Gita: The Complete Bhagavad Gita — A Commentary for Modern Readers*. Henry Holt and Co., Inc., 1990

Satchinananda, Sri Swami. *Yoga Sutras of Pantanjali*. Inner Traditions International. Vermont, USA, 1989

Smith, Houston. *The Illustrated World's Religions: A Guide to Our Wisdom Traditions*. Harpers. San Francisco, 1991

Svatmarama, Swami. *Hathayoga Pradipika*. Commentary by Hans Ulrich Reiker. Aquarian Press, 1992

Usharbudh, Arya. *Philosophy of Hatha Yoga*. Himalayan Inst Pr, 1985

index

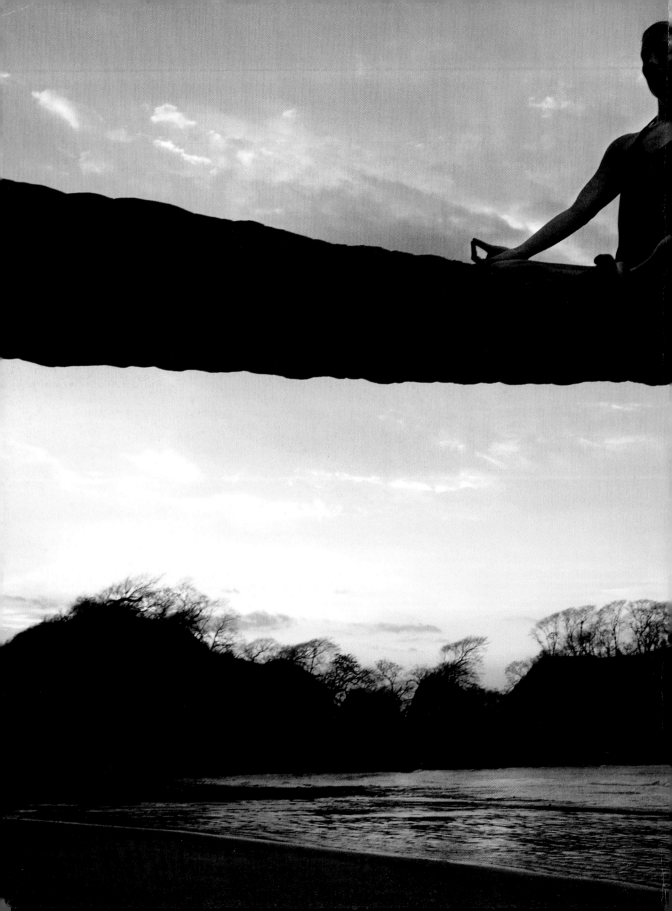

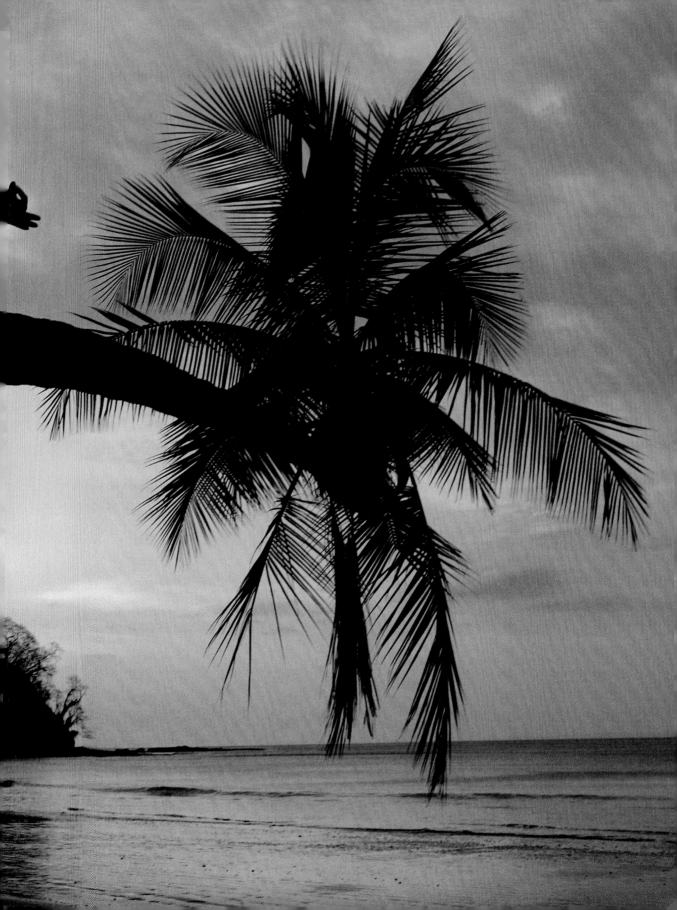